T0263296

Small Animal Obesity

Editors

AMY K. FARCAS
KATHRYN E. MICHEL

VETERINARY CLINICS OF NORTH AMERICA: SMALL ANIMAL PRACTICE

www.vetsmall.theclinics.com

September 2016 • Volume 46 • Number 5

ELSEVIER

1600 John F. Kennedy Boulevard • Suite 1800 • Philadelphia, Pennsylvania, 19103-2899
http://www.vetsmall.theclinics.com

VETERINARY CLINICS OF NORTH AMERICA: SMALL ANIMAL PRACTICE Volume 46, Number 5
September 2016 ISSN 0195-5616, ISBN-13: 978-0-323-46270-9

Editor: Patrick Manley
Developmental Editor: Meredith Clinton

Veterinary Clinics of North America: Small Animal Practice (ISSN 0195-5616) is published bimonthly by Elsevier Inc., 360 Park Avenue South, New York, NY 10010-1710. Months of issue are January, March, May, July, September, and November. Business and Editorial Offices: 1600 John F. Kennedy Blvd., Ste. 1800, Philadelphia, PA 19103-2899. Customer Service Office: 3251 Riverport Lane, Maryland Heights, MO 63043. Periodicals postage paid at New York, NY and additional mailing offices. Subscription prices are $310.00 per year (domestic individuals), $564.00 per year (domestic institutions), $100.00 per year (domestic students/residents), $410.00 per year (Canadian individuals), $701.00 per year (Canadian institutions), $455.00 per year (international individuals), $701.00 per year (international institutions), and $220.00 per year (international and Canadian students/residents). To receive student/resident rate, orders must be accompanied by name of affiliated institution, date of term, and the *signature* of program/residency coordinator on institution letterhead. Orders will be billed at individual rate until proof of status is received. Foreign air speed delivery is included in all *Clinics* subscription prices. All prices are subject to change without notice. **POSTMASTER:** Send address changes to *Veterinary Clinics of North America: Small Animal Practice*, Elsevier Health Sciences Division, Subscription Customer Service, 3251 Riverport Lane, Maryland Heights, MO 63043. Customer Service (orders, claims, online, change of address): Elsevier Periodicals Customer Service, Elsevier Health Sciences Division Subscription **Customer Service 3251 Riverport Lane Maryland Heights, MO 63043. Tel: 1-800-654-2452 (U.S. and Canada); 314-447-8871 (outside U.S. and Canada). Fax: 314-447-8029. E-mail: journalscustomerservice-usa@elsevier.com (for print support); journalsonlinesupport-usa@elsevier.com (for online support).**

Reprints. For copies of 100 or more of articles in this publication, please contact the Commercial Reprints Department, Elsevier Inc., 360 Park Avenue South, New York, NY 10010-1710. Tel.: 212-633-3874; Fax: 212-633-3820; E-mail: reprints@elsevier.com.

Veterinary Clinics of North America: Small Animal Practice is also published in Japanese by Inter Zoo Publishing Co., Ltd., Aoyama Crystal-Bldg 5F, 3-5-12 Kitaaoyama, Minato-ku, Tokyo 107-0061, Japan.

Veterinary Clinics of North America: Small Animal Practice is covered in *Current Contents/Agriculture, Biology and Environmental Sciences, Science Citation Index, ASCA, MEDLINE/PubMed (Index Medicus), Excerpta Medica, and BIOSIS.*

Contributors

EDITORS

AMY K. FARCAS, DVM, MS, DACVN
Owner, Veterinary Nutritionist, Veterinary Nutrition Care, San Carlos, California

KATHRYN E. MICHEL, DVM, MS, MSED, DACVN
Professor of Nutrition, Department of Clinical Studies—Philadelphia, School of Veterinary Medicine, University of Pennsylvania, Philadelphia, Pennsylvania

AUTHORS

ROBERT BACKUS, MS, DVM, PhD
Diplomate, American College of Veterinary Nutrition; Associate Professor and Director of the Nestlé Purina Endowed Program in Small Animal Nutrition, Department of Veterinary Medicine and Surgery, University of Missouri College of Veterinary Medicine, Columbia, Missouri

MARJORIE L. CHANDLER, DVM, MS, MANZCVS, MRCVS
Diplomate, American College of Veterinary Nutrition; Diplomate, American College of Veterinary Internal Medicine; Diplomate, European College of Veterinary Internal Medicine – Small Animal; Clinical Nutritionist, Vets Now Referrals, Glasgow, Scotland

JULIE CHURCHILL, DVM, PhD
Diplomate, American College of Veterinary Nutrition; Board Member of Pet Nutrition Alliance; Board Member of Association for Pet Obesity Prevention; Associate Professor of Veterinary Nutrition, Department of Veterinary Clinical Sciences, University of Minnesota College of Veterinary Medicine, Saint Paul, Minnesota

MELISSA CLARK, DVM, PhD
Diplomate, American College of Veterinary Clinical Pharmacology; Resident, Department of Internal Medicine, The Animal Medical Center, New York, New York

LAURA EIRMANN, DVM
Diplomate, American College of Veterinary Nutrition; Clinical Nutritionist, Nutrition Service, Oradell Animal Hospital, Paramus, New Jersey; Manager, Veterinary Communications, Nestlé Purina PetCare, St Louis, Missouri

CHRISTOPHER W. FRYE, DVM
Department of Clinical Sciences, Cornell University College of Veterinary Medicine, Ithaca, New York

ALEXANDER JAMES GERMAN, BVSc(Hons), PhD
Institute of Ageing and Chronic Disease; Institute of Veterinary Sciences, University of Liverpool, Neston, Merseyside, United Kingdom

BETH HAMPER, DVM, PhD
Diplomate, American College of Veterinary Nutrition; Hamper Veterinary Nutritional Consulting, Indianapolis, Indiana

MARGARETHE HOENIG, DVM, PhD, Dr med vet
Professor, Department of Veterinary Clinical Medicine, College of Veterinary Medicine, University of Illinois at Urbana-Champaign, Urbana-Champaign, Illinois

JENNIFER A. LARSEN, DVM, PhD
Diplomate, American College of Veterinary Nutrition; Associate Professor of Clinical Nutrition, VM: Molecular Biosciences, School of Veterinary Medicine, University of California, Davis, Davis, California

DEBORAH E. LINDER, DVM
Diplomate, American College of Veterinary Nutrition; Research Assistant Professor, Department of Clinical Sciences, Cummings School of Veterinary Medicine at Tufts University, North Grafton, Massachusetts

MARYANNE MURPHY, DVM, PhD
Diplomate, American College of Veterinary Nutrition; Department of Clinical Nutrition, Red Bank Veterinary Hospital, Tinton Falls, New Jersey

VALERIE J. PARKER, DVM
Diplomate, American College of Veterinary Internal Medicine; Diplomate, American College of Veterinary Nutrition; Assistant Professor – Clinical, Department of Veterinary Clinical Sciences, The Ohio State University, Columbus, Ohio

JUSTIN W. SHMALBERG, DVM
Diplomate, American College of Veterinary Sports Medicine and Rehabilitation; Diplomate, American College of Veterinary Nutrition; Department of Clinical Sciences, University of Florida College of Veterinary Medicine, Gainesville, Florida

CECILIA VILLAVERDE, BVSc, PhD
Diplomate, American College of Veterinary Nutrition; Diplomate, European College of Veterinary and Comparative Nutrition; Departament de Ciència Animal i dels Aliments (Animal and Food Science Department), Universitat Autònoma de Barcelona, Bellaterra, Spain

JOSEPH J. WAKSHLAG, DVM, PhD
Diplomate, American College of Veterinary Sports Medicine and Rehabilitation; Diplomate, American College of Veterinary Nutrition; Department of Clinical Sciences, Cornell University College of Veterinary Medicine, Ithaca, New York

ALLISON WARA, DVM
Clinical Instructor of Veterinary Nutrition and Director of the Small Animal Physical Rehabilitation and Nutrition Clinic, Department of Veterinary Medicine and Surgery, University of Missouri College of Veterinary Medicine, Columbia, Missouri

ERNIE WARD, DVM, CVFT
Founder, Association for Pet Obesity Prevention, E3 Management, LLC, Ocean Isle Beach, North Carolina

LISA P. WEETH, DVM, MRCVS
Diplomate, American College of Veterinary Nutrition; Veterinary Clinical Nutritionist, Weeth Nutrition Services, Edinburgh, United Kingdom; Clinical Nutrition Department, Telemedicine Services, Gulf Coast Veterinary Specialists, Houston, Texas

Contents

> Obesity is a common disease of modern dogs and cats. Dog and cat owners often do not realize their animal is affected. Some pet owners are skeptical of the diagnosis or rationalize the overweight condition of their pets. Animal-related factors associated with obesity in dogs and cats include breed, neuter status, age, and gender, whereas owner-related factors include diet choice, feeding method, and provision of exercise. Owner characteristics, such as age and income, are also potential risk factors for pet obesity. Identifying such risk factors for both animals and owners may help provide targets for prevention or interventional tools.

> Normal adult animals living in nonstressful environments that receive nutritionally sound diets balance their energy expenditure with their energy intake over the long-term. Most knowledge of mechanisms underlying the precise balance of energy is derived from research on rodent models and human correlates. This knowledge is believed to be applicable and pertinent for understanding causes of obesity in dogs and cats. The roles of satiation and adiposity feedback, cognitive input, energy expenditure, and physical activity are reviewed. Dietary and environmental factors especially relevant to promotion of overweight body condition are reviewed. These include dietary fat and palatability, inactive and stressful lifestyle, and obesogenic effects of neutering.

> The domestication and urbanization of dogs and cats has dramatically altered their environment and behavior. Human and pet obesity is a global concern, particularly in developed countries. An increased incidence of chronic disease is associated with obesity secondary to low-grade systemic inflammation. This article reviews current research into the genetic, dietary, and physiologic factors associated with obesity, along with use of "omics" technology to better understand and characterize this disease.

> Obesity in pet dogs and cats is a significant problem in developed countries, and seems to be increasing in prevalence. Excess body fat has

adverse metabolic consequences, including insulin resistance, altered adipokine secretion, changes in metabolic rate, abnormal lipid metabolism, and fat accumulation in visceral organs. Obese cats are predisposed to endocrine and metabolic disorders such as diabetes and hepatic lipidosis. A connection likely also exists between obesity and diabetes mellitus in dogs. No system has been developed to identify obese pets at greatest risk for development of obesity-associated metabolic diseases, and further study in this area is needed.

Although there are known detrimental effects of obesity on the heart and lungs, few data exist showing obesity as a risk factor for cardiopulmonary disorders in dogs and cats. It is probable that increased abdominal fat is detrimental, as it is in humans, and there is evidence of negative effects of increased intrathoracic fat. In addition to the physical effects of fat, increased inflammatory mediators and neurohormonal effects of obesity likely contribute to cardiopulmonary disorders, as well. Weight loss in overweight individuals improves cardiac parameters and exercise tolerance. Obesity in patients with obstructive airway disorders is recognized to increase disease severity.

Osteoarthritis is common among aging canine and feline patients. The incidence and severity of clinical lameness are closely correlated to body condition in overweight and obese patients. Excessive adiposity may result in incongruous and excessive mechanical loading that worsens clinical signs in affected patients. Data suggest a potential link between adipokines, obesity-related inflammation, and a worsening of the underlying pathology. Similarly, abnormal physical stress and generalized systemic inflammation propagated by obesity contribute to neurologic signs associated with intervertebral disc disease. Weight loss and exercise are critical to ameliorating the pain and impaired mobility of affected animals.

Obesity is not a cosmetic or social issue; it is an animal health issue. The metabolic effects of obesity on insulin resistance and development of hyperlipidemia and the mechanical stress excess weight places on the musculoskeletal system are well established in the literature. Additional health risks from obesity, such as fatty accumulation in the liver, intestinal bacterial dysbiosis, and changes to renal architecture, are less well understood, but have been demonstrated to occur clinically in obese animals and may lead to deleterious long-term health effects. Keeping dogs and cats lean lowers their risk for development of certain diseases and leads to a longer and better quality of life.

> Nutritional assessment focuses on evaluation of animal-specific, diet-specific, feeding management, and environmental factors. Assessment includes evaluation of a patient's medical history, comprehensive diet history, and physical examination including body weight, body condition, and muscle condition. Diagnostic testing may identify comorbidities associated with obesity or concurrent health conditions that need to be considered when developing a nutrition plan. When obesity is diagnosed during the nutritional assessment this finding along with health implications must be clearly communicated to the pet owner. Careful consideration of animal-specific, diet-specific, owner-specific, and environmental factors allows the clinician to develop a specific nutrition plan tailored to the needs of pet and owner.

> The optimal weight loss diet for cats and dogs is best determined by obtaining a full dietary history and performing a detailed assessment of the pet, pet owner, and environment in which the pet lives. Incorporating information about pet and owner preferences allows for individualization of the weight management plan and has the potential to increase adherence. Calorie density, macronutrients, and micronutrient concentrations should be considered as part of a weight management plan. Owners should play an active role in the weight loss plan to have the best outcome.

> Obesity is commonly encountered in veterinary patients. Although there are various published dietary approaches to achieving weight loss, successful long-term prevention of weight regain has proven elusive. Adding environmental and behavioral treatment strategies to a weight loss plan may help the veterinary team, the pet, and the pet owner maximize the effectiveness of the program. Because the owner directly affects the environment and behavior of the pet undergoing a weight loss plan, treatment strategies with an emphasis on owner involvement is the focus of this review. Veterinary use of the 5 A's behavioral counseling approach with the pet owner is discussed.

> Obesity continues to be the most prevalent nutritional problem of dogs and cats as well as one of the most frustrating conditions to treat successfully. Educating and assigning roles to all members of the health care team will improve staff engagement and the consistency and effectiveness of

nutritional counseling for preventive care and weight loss treatment plans. Excellent communication skills can be used to assess the client's ability to change and implement a weight loss plan at the right time in the right way to achieve better adherence and improve patient health.

Alexander James German

Obesity is one of the most prevalent medical diseases in pets. Outcomes are often disappointing; many animals either fail to reach target weight, or regain weight. This article discusses managing obesity and focusing on prevention. It gives guidance on establishing monitoring programs that use regular body weight and condition assessments to identify animals at risk of inappropriate weight gain, enabling early intervention. Weight management in obese animals is a lifelong process. Regular weight and body condition monitoring are key to identifying animals that rebound early, while continuing to feed a therapeutic weight loss diet can help prevent it from happening.

VETERINARY CLINICS OF NORTH AMERICA: SMALL ANIMAL PRACTICE

THE CLINICS ARE NOW AVAILABLE ONLINE!
Access your subscription at:
www.theclinics.com

Preface

Confronting the Problem of Obesity in Dogs and Cats

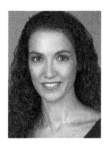 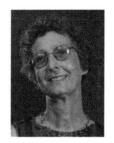

Amy K. Farcas, DVM, MS, DACVN   Kathryn E. Michel, DVM, MS, MSED, DACVN

Editors

It has been over 20 years since Lund and colleagues[1] collected data on more than 30,000 dogs and 14,000 cats seen at primary care practices throughout the United States. This large-scale investigation revealed that approximately 28% of dogs and cats were identified as overweight or obese. Since then, the problem of obesity in companion animals has been the focus of a substantial number of investigations ranging from epidemiologic studies of risk factors to controlled trials in a laboratory or clinical setting to bench-top research in areas such as genetics, omics, and the microbiome. Addressing obesity in dogs and cats has also garnered attention in the private sector, including the development of over-the-counter and therapeutic pet foods, pharmaceuticals, and a range of products designed to control food intake, promote exercise, or provide environmental enrichment.

Despite all of this attention, the problem of pet dog and cat obesity is still with us. Moreover, recent studies document an even greater prevalence of overweight and obesity in companion animals, and not just in the United States, but also worldwide. It is becoming clear that confronting this problem will likely require a change in how both pet owners and veterinarians think about it.

Obesity is more than just a cosmetic issue. Adipose tissue is an organ by definition, and obesity is now recognized as, and should be presented to pet owners in the context of, organ dysfunction. Excess weight should be included in a patient's problem list, just as cardiac or kidney dysfunction would be, so that a plan can be made to address it. Furthermore, as with any form of organ dysfunction, adipose tissue dysfunction can contribute to diseases of other organs and systems.

To be the best advocates for their patients, veterinarians will need to effectively convey that, contrary to popular belief, overweight/obesity is not normal and needs to be addressed appropriately.

We recognize that the problem of obesity is not an easy one to discuss with pet owners, to prevent, to treat, or to manage, and it is our hope that this issue of the

Vet Clin Small Anim 46 (2016) xi–xii
http://dx.doi.org/10.1016/j.cvsm.2016.06.015
0195-5616/16/$ – see front matter © 2016 Published by Elsevier Inc.
vetsmall.theclinics.com

Veterinary Clinics of North America: Small Animal Practice will help to overcome these challenges. We have endeavored to bring together experts in the research on and the clinical management of the problem of obesity in dogs and cats to provide a current and comprehensive review encompassing pathogenesis, risk factors, health consequences, and available therapeutic interventions, including diet, exercise, and behavioral modification. It is our hope that it will be an essential resource for the small animal practitioner who serves in the frontline for the prevention and treatment of this serious condition.

Amy K. Farcas, DVM, MS, DACVN
Owner, Veterinary Nutritionist
Veterinary Nutrition Care
987 Laurel Street
San Carlos, CA 94070, USA

Kathryn E. Michel, DVM, MS, MSED, DACVN
Professor of Nutrition
Department of Clinical Studies—Philadelphia
School of Veterinary Medicine
University of Pennsylvania
M.J. Ryan VHUP
3900 Delancey Street
Philadelphia, PA 19104-6010, USA

E-mail addresses:
amy@veterinarynutritioncare.com (A.K. Farcas)
michel@vet.upenn.edu (K.E. Michel)

REFERENCE

1. Lund EM, Armstrong PJ, Kirk CA, et al. Health status and population characteristics of dogs and cats examined at private veterinary practices in the United States. J Am Vet Med Assoc 1999;214(9):1336–41.

Scope of the Problem and Perception by Owners and Veterinarians

Jennifer A. Larsen, DVM, PhD[a],*, Cecilia Villaverde, BVSc, PhD[b]

KEYWORDS

• Feeding • Feline • Canine • Obesity • Diet • Nutrition

KEY POINTS

- Obesity is a common disease of dogs and cats, affecting well over half of the animals in some populations.
- Many owners apparently do not recognize obesity in their dogs and cats and tend to rationalize or justify the problem with humanization of the pet.
- The presence of obesity in dogs and cats is associated with both animal factors (such as breed and neuter status) and owner factors (such as diet choice and provision of exercise).

INTRODUCTION

Obesity is one of the most common and most important chronic diseases in dogs and cats and is associated with a variety of disease conditions as well as shortened life span. Although the scope and impact of this problem have been described in different populations, and the benefits of a lean body condition are reported, obesity remains a frustratingly difficult condition to reverse. In addition, successful weight loss is often not maintained, with many pets regaining weight in a short time. The vital roles of the veterinarian and pet owner in preventing obesity, or in recognizing and successfully addressing it once it occurs, cannot be underestimated.

EPIDEMIOLOGY
Disease Description

Body condition scoring (BCS) systems are an invaluable tool in the assessment of all patients. In obese pets, the BCS can be used to diagnose obesity and to monitor a

Dr J.A. Larsen has nothing to disclose. Dr C. Villaverde is a consultant for various pet food companies.
[a] VM: Molecular Biosciences, School of Veterinary Medicine, University of California, Davis, One Shields Avenue, Davis, CA 95616, USA; [b] Departament de Ciència Animal i dels Aliments (Animal and Food Science Department), Universitat Autònoma de Barcelona, Edifici V, Campus UAB, Bellaterra 08193, Spain
* Corresponding author.
E-mail address: jalarsen@vmth.ucdavis.edu

patient during weight loss. Although subjective, this provides a quantitative way to estimate the amount of excess adipose present and the ideal body weight. Using the 9-point system (which has been validated using more objective measures of adiposity), each point represents 10% to 5% of body weight.[1,2] Obesity is defined, as in people, as weighing approximately 25% or more over ideal, which is equivalent to 7 or more on a 9-point scale. Adverse effects of obesity in dogs and cats affect many different body systems and may include exacerbations of orthopedic, dermatologic, and cardiopulmonary diseases; insulin resistance and diabetes mellitus; altered hemostasis; hepatic lipidosis; and shortened life span.[3–12] (See Melissa Clark and Margarethe Hoenig's article, "Metabolic Effects of Obesity and Its Interaction with Endocrine Diseases"; Marjorie L. Chandler's article, "Impact of Obesity on Cardiopulmonary Disease"; Christopher W. Frye, Justin W. Shmalberg, and Joseph J. Wakshlag's article, "Obesity, Exercise and Orthopedic Disease"; and Lisa P. Weeth's article, "Other Risks/Possible Benefits of Obesity," in this issue.)

Prevalence

Obesity is a common and serious problem in domestic dogs and cats. Studies have reported that some cat populations have a prevalence of overweight and obese cats of up to 63% (**Table 1**).[3,13–19] Similarly, prevalence of overweight and obesity in various populations of dogs reportedly range up to 59.3% (**Table 2**).[12,20–26]

OWNER PERCEPTIONS

Recognition and acknowledgment of obesity by both the owner and the veterinary team are critical to effectively address the problem. To achieve success in any weight

Table 1				
Selected reported prevalences of veterinary-diagnosed feline overweight and obesity				
Reference	Geographic Location	n	Prevalence	Risk Factors and Associations
Scarlett et al,[13] 1994	Northeast US veterinary clinics	>2000	24%	Indoor living, inactivity, middle age, male, neuter, mixed breed, some dry foods
Russell et al,[14] 2000	London (UK) households	136	52%	Neuter, middle age, frequent treating, free feeding
Lund et al,[3] 2005	US veterinary clinics	8159	35%	Neuter, male, premium or therapeutic food, breed
Colliard et al,[15] 2009	National Veterinary School of Alfort teaching hospital (Paris, France)	385	26.8%	Male, neuter, owners underestimating BCS
Courcier et al,[16] 2010	Glasgow, Scotland	118	39%	Frequency of feeding, neutered status
Cave et al,[17] 2012	Households urban area (Palmerston North, New Zealand)	200	63%	Age, longer leg length, owners underestimating BCS
Courcier et al,[18] 2012	Great Britain veterinary clinics	3227	11.5%	Neuter status, male, middle age
Corbee,[19] 2014	Show cats in the Netherlands	268	45.5%	Neuter status, breed

Table 2
Selected reported prevalences of veterinary-diagnosed canine overweight and obesity

Reference	Geographic Location	n	Prevalence	Risk Factors and Associations
Kronfeld et al,[20] 1991	Veterinary Hospital of the University of Pennsylvania	3729	22.9%	Breed, middle age
McGreevy et al,[21] 2005	Veterinary practices in Australia	2661	41.1%	Middle age, neuter, breed, female, rural and semirural region
Lund et al,[12] 2006	US veterinary clinics	21,754	34%	Neuter, age, semimoist, canned, or homemade food, consumption of table scraps or commercial treats, breed, geographic region
Colliard et al,[22] 2006	National Veterinary School of Alfort teaching hospital (Paris, France)	616	38.8%	Neuter, female, age, breed, older or retired owner, homemade food
Weeth et al,[23] 2007	Veterinary Medical Teaching Hospital of University of California, Davis	14,670	36.4%	Neuter, breed
Courcier et al,[24] 2010	Veterinary practices in UK	696	59.3%	Frequency of snacks/treats, increasing owner age and lower income, hours weekly exercise
Corbee,[25] 2013	Show dogs in the Netherlands	1379	18.6%	Certain breed groups
Mao et al,[26] 2013	China	2391	44.4%	Noncommercial food, neuter, female, middle age, low activity, feeding more than once per day

loss program, an owner must alter often long-standing feeding practices and habits. To change these factors, an understanding of the benefits of weight loss as well as the importance of both reversing the overweight condition and maintaining a lean conformation is valuable. Unfortunately, many owners do not recognize obesity in their pets.

Many studies have shown that owners have unrealistic perceptions of the body condition of their dogs[22,27–29] and cats.[15,17,30] This underestimation may have an impact on whether the owner choses to pursue a weight loss program and may actually contribute to the development of obesity in the first place. Therefore, underestimation of body condition by the owner seems an important risk factor for pet obesity.

In addition, 1 study reported the important observation that owners tended to justify obesity in their dogs by providing explanations regarding alleged improvement or by humanizing and relating to a pet's desire for treats.[27] For many families, feeding and treating may be a way to show affection and attention to a pet. Also, some owners were skeptical of the diagnosis,[27] which may be a defense mechanism to deny a perceived accusation that they have done something harmful when informed of health risks and potential adverse outcomes associated with their pet's obesity. Furthermore, in the authors' experience, some owners assert that they believe food restriction would cause their pet to suffer and that they instead would prefer that their pets are "happy" even if overweight and with a shorter life span. This may also be a way to justify a pet's condition as well as rationalize their lack of intent to address the problem. However, one recent study found that overweight cats subjected to weight loss were actually reportedly more affectionate than before the plan started, even though their food seeking behavior also increased.[31]

Together with owner recognition and understanding of the problem, effective client communication is critical to ensuring this understanding and helping achieve a successful weight loss program. Some clinicians are reluctant, however, to discuss pet obesity and the associated health problems, in particular with owners who may also be overweight. Under these circumstances, an effective weight loss solution will never be achieved. Clinicians should not be reluctant to diagnose an overweight condition in any pet and should initiate a dialog to ensure that owners understand that their pet is overweight as well as the importance of reversing the condition. (See Julie Churchill and Ernie Ward's article, "Communicating with Pet Owners About Obesity: Roles of the Veterinary Health Care Team," in this issue.)

CAUSES/PREDISPOSITIONS FOR OBESITY

Obesity ultimately results from an imbalance between energy intake and energy expenditure, and the different causative factors can influence 1 or both sides of the energy balance. Several epidemiologic studies (see **Tables 1** and **2**) have identified associations and risk factors for obesity in both dogs and cats (**Box 1**). Not all studies identify the same factors, however, which underscores the need for prospective studies that may elucidate any causal relationships.

Animal Factors

Breed

Some breeds of dogs and cats are at higher risk for developing obesity, and this genetic predisposition seems to result in higher BCS in some populations (**Box 2**).[3,12,19,21,22,25,32]

Two studies from Corbee[19,25] assessing BCS in dogs and cats that were competing at shows in the Netherlands demonstrated strong breed predispositions and a high prevalence of overweight animals in these events (18.6% for dogs and 45.5% for cats), which might indicate that some breed standards promote a BCS considered too high relative to those determined ideal for reducing morbidity due to a variety of diseases.[19,25]

Box 1
Factors associated with overweight and obesity in dogs and cats

- Animal factors
  - Breed
  - Gender
  - Neuter status (sterilization)
  - Growth rate
  - Age
- Owner factors
  - Diet choice
  - Feeding method
  - Exercise and living environment
  - Age and body composition of owner
  - Income
  - Underestimation of pet's BCS

| **Box 2** |
| **Dog and cat breeds at higher risk of obesity** |

Dogs

- Labrador retriever
- Golden retriever
- Cocker spaniel
- Dachshund
- Dalmatian
- Rottweiler
- Shetland sheepdog

Cats

- Domestic short hair
- Domestic medium hair
- Domestic long hair
- Manx
- British short hair
- Norwegian forest cat
- Persian

The reason for the increased risk of obesity in certain breeds may be related to lower energy needs. The wide range of body sizes in the canine species in particular results in an effect of allometry of energy requirements and may partly explain some breed variation.[33] Even within similar sizes, however, breed variation in energy needs has been reported.[34,35] Two meta-analyses, 1 in cats[36] and 1 in dogs,[37] failed to find an effect of breed on maintenance energy requirements in adult animals. It is also possible that in some cases the drive to eat or general interest in food is higher than seen in other dogs or cats, even though there is little information about this aspect. One recent article proposed a questionnaire to evaluate this in dogs, using a "food motivation core," inspired by questionnaires used for children.[38] When they applied the questionnaire to a population of dogs, they found that this score was positively correlated to BCS, thus potentially linking this drive to eat with increased difficulty for owners in limiting access to food. The same study also found that owners of overweight dogs exerted more control over how they fed their pets compared with owners of lean dogs, indicating that these owners, up to a point, were aware that their pets needed feeding management. An epidemiologic study also found that owner-reported "good appetite" was associated with a higher BCS in dogs.[39]

Gender
Some feline studies have identified being male as a risk factor for obesity,[3,13,15] although others have not (see **Table 1**). On the other hand, most studies in dogs did not report a gender association although some identified being female as a risk factor.[21,22,26]

Sterilization
The practice of neutering pets is linked to known effects on physiology and behavior that predispose to obesity, which is the most significant sequela from a nutritional

perspective. Neutering has been consistently associated with an increased risk of obesity in pet dogs and cats[15,16,18,21,40–42] and is also associated with a lower energy requirement in both cats and dogs.[36,37]

The relationships among food intake, body weight and condition, and energy expenditure are complex. It seems clear, however, that when cats are free fed, especially after neutering, weight gain is likely to occur[43–46]; and free availability of food results in greater body weight and body fat percentage after neutering of male cats as well as female cats compared with restricted access.[47,48] This effect is even seen in feral cats participating in trap-neuter-release programs.[49] In addition, greater weight gains and body fat accumulation are seen after neutering when energy dense diets are used.[50,51]

Regarding dogs, there is much less information. One study following mixed breed dogs after early (7 weeks) or later (7 months) gonadectomy did not find any differences in food intake, weight gain, or back fat depth.[52] A more recent study, although with a low number of kennel dogs, found that sterilization of female dogs resulted in a decrease in energy expenditure (estimated by energy intake needed to maintain a stable body weight).[53] Moreover, free feeding these spayed dogs resulted in an increase in food intake, which resulted in weight gain. Overall, these results suggest that portion control is important to prevent undesired weight gain in sterilized pets.

Growth rate

One study of colony cats that were free fed found that growth rate in kittens was strongly associated with being overweight as an adult.[54] This suggests that prevention needs to start early in life, independently of the neuter status of the cats.

Age

Obesity is considered a disease of the middle aged, both in cats[13,14,17] and in dogs.[12,21]

Owner Factors

Owner factors relate to the relationship between owners and pets, including diet choice, feeding method, provision of environment and exercise, and all other aspects of the human-animal bond. Owner behavior relating to feeding management plays a large role in the body condition of pets as reviewed by Linder and Mueller.[55]

Diet choice

Trends in pet food marketing and formulation must also be considered. Palatability, energy density, and label feeding directions may all contribute to overfeeding of and overconsumption by pets. Manufacturers of pet foods aim to produce palatable diets that are enthusiastically accepted and quickly eaten, because this reinforces to the consumer that the diet selected is well liked by their pet. Palatability, however, may supersede satiety for many pets. Palatable diets that are also energy dense (because they are typically high in fat) may contribute to overconsumption of energy and inappropriate weight gain.

In cats, the feeding of therapeutic diets (those available from veterinarians and intended to prevent or treat a disease) and premium diets (those available from veterinary clinics or small and large pet stores) was reported to be associated with overweight and obesity; the investigators of that study speculated that this was due to the typically higher energy density of such diets.[3] Another epidemiologic study also found therapeutic diets were a risk factor in cats.[13] One prospective study evaluating cats at approximately 3, 7, and 12 months of age in the United Kingdom identified 2 risk factors for being reported overweight by the owner at 1 year of age: 1 that the main diet fed was dry and the other that the cat had limited access to the outdoors.[56] Although the number of cats included in that study was large (966), only 7% of the cats included were overweight. In addition, owner-reported BCS can be inaccurate.[29] Another limitation that may influence interpretation of this investigation was that the owners were not asked about the type of dry diet used (marketing category, life stage, price point, and so forth).[56] This might be important because 1 study found that feeding a diet not adequate for growth to kittens was associated with obesity in adult cats,[42] and another identified specific food types (premium or therapeutic diets) as risk factors for obesity.[3] Not all epidemiologic studies, however, have found the type of diet a risk factor for feline obesity.[15,17,30]

Similarly, not all studies have identified the type of diet as a risk factor for canine obesity. Two studies have found an association, however, between dogs fed home-prepared diets and being overweight.[22,26] Another study from the United States also found an association with obesity and feeding homemade and canned diets, and the investigators proposed that the energy density of these foods could contribute to obesity.[12]

Feeding method

Together with palatable, energy-dense diets, the lack of guidance available for pet owners with regard to the individualized energy needs of their pet may contribute to obesity. There are well documented challenges in determination of energy requirements of populations and individuals.[57] There is some evidence that feeding directions on pet food labels are inaccurate and often overestimate energy needs, especially for neutered adult pets.[58] Label feeding directions are based on estimates of energy requirements of healthy laboratory dogs and cats that are in normal body condition, undertake little to modest amounts of physical activity, and in a controlled thermoneutral environment. In addition, the determination and reporting of metabolizable energy (ME) in pet foods is not always accurate.[59] The ME content of pet food can be determined either experimentally or by using formulas (such as the one published by the National Research Council in 2006,[60] among others). This can result in widely variable ME contents of pet foods, which contributes to the inaccuracy of label instructions. In some countries, the ME content of pet foods is not even reported in the label, although in the United States this became compulsory in 2014.

Feeding table scraps and excessive treating have been identified as risk factors for obesity, primarily in dogs,[12,22,24,38,39,61–63] although 1 study[14] also identified this in cats. Treating can contribute significantly to excessive energy intake and could potentially interfere with weight loss plans, although 1 study in the United Kingdom did not find that a history of owner treating affected the success of the weight loss program.[64]

Information regarding the role of meal frequency is less clear. In dogs, 1 study demonstrated that owners of obese dogs were more likely to feed 1 meal per day or 3 or more meals per day versus 2 meals per day.[61] A different study also identified feeding once a day as a risk factor,[62] although another[63] found that owners of obese dogs were more likely to feed multiple meals per day, whereas Mao and colleagues[26] found that feeding once a day was protective. For cats, although only 1 epidemiologic study in cats found that free feeding was associated with a high BCS,[14] several prospective experimental studies support that free feeding, especially of neutered cats, can result in unwanted weight gain.[43–46]

Exercise and living environment

Indoor living (or restricted outdoor access) has been associated with high BCS in cats in both epidemiologic and prospective studies, presumably due to restricted activity.[13,42,56] Higher physical activity and exercise have been shown to reduce obesity risk in dogs in several retrospective studies as well,[24,26,38,61,62] and owners of obese dogs are more likely to rely on dogs self-exercising in their yard rather than walking them.[61] One study in medium to large breed dogs assessed activity 3 times over 10 weeks and found an inverse correlation between BCS and number of steps, supporting the positive effect of exercise on body condition in dogs.[65]

Because exercise seems important in preventing obesity, Degeling and colleagues[66] aimed to study the owner factors that result in dogs getting adequate exercise (determined as more than 150 minutes per week). This study found that housing determined the frequency of walks but not total minutes of exercise, where owners living in apartments walked their dogs more frequently compared with owners living in houses. This could be related to the lack of a backyard (and thus greater need for walks for elimination) or to a social environment that promotes walking dogs. This study also identified that dog breeds that were characterized by the British Kennel Club as having higher exercise requirements were walked more minutes than other breeds, even though most dogs walked fewer minutes than the recommendations of the British Kennel Club.[66]

Owner characteristics

Some studies have found that obese dogs are more likely to have older[22,24,67] or obese[63] owners but similar findings have not been confirmed in cats.[68] Kienzle and colleagues[63] have also reported that owners of obese dogs speak more to their pets, are more likely to allow their pets to sleep with them, and spend more time watching their pets eat, leading these investigators to hypothesize that owners of obese dogs might be more likely to "humanize" their pets. This same study also identified that owners of obese pets had lower income and spent less money on their pet's food.[63] Likewise, Courcier and colleagues[24] also identified lower family income as a risk factor for canine obesity, and Suarez and colleagues[67] reported that owners of overweight dogs were more sensitive to low prices and sales compared with those of normal-weight dogs.

Finally, another owner characteristic that has been identified in both canine[22] and feline[15,17,30] studies as risky is that owners underestimate their pet's BCS. Courcier and colleagues[29] evaluated a population of dogs in Glasgow, United Kingdom, and compared BCS given by owners and by veterinarians and found that 44% of owners underestimated their dog's BCS.

SUMMARY

In summary, there are many factors that can favor the development of overweight and obesity in dogs and cats, and owner-related factors, such as diet choice, feeding methods and practices, and environment, are important and need to be addressed in all dogs and cats to prevent (and reverse) obesity. Ultimately, evidence supports avoidance of free feeding, consideration for diet energy density, provision of a life stage–appropriate diet, and regular monitoring of the body condition of neutered pets. Determination of energy needs should be based on prior intake, if known; however, the degree of restriction necessary to avoid weight gain is variable and underscores the importance of monitoring and adjustment.

REFERENCES

1. Laflamme D. Development and validation of a body condition score system for cats: a clinical tool. Feline Practice 1997;25:13–8.
2. Laflamme DP. Development and validation of a body condition score system for dogs. Canine Practice 1997;22:10–5.

3. Lund EM, Armstrong PJ, Kirk CA, et al. Prevalence and risk factors for obesity in adult cats from private US veterinary practices. Int J Appl Res Vet Med 2005;3: 88–96.
4. Bjornvad CR, Wiinberg B, Kristensen AT. Obesity increases initial rate of fibrin formation during blood coagulation in domestic shorthaired cats. J Anim Physiol Anim Nutr (Berl) 2012;96:834–41.
5. Scarlett JM, Donoghue S. Associations between body condition and disease in cats. J Am Vet Med Assoc 1998;212:1725–31.
6. Kealy RD, Lawler DF, Ballam JM, et al. Evaluation of the effect of limited food consumption on radiographic evidence of osteoarthritis in dogs. J Am Vet Med Assoc 2000;217:1678–80.
7. Kealy RD, Lawler DF, Ballam JM, et al. Effects of diet restriction on life span and age-related changes in dogs. J Am Vet Med Assoc 2002;220:1315–20.
8. Larson BT, Lawler DF, Spitznagel EL Jr, et al. Improved glucose tolerance with lifetime diet restriction favorably affects disease and survival in dogs. J Nutr 2003;133:2887–92.
9. Lawler DF, Evans RH, Larson BT, et al. Influence of lifetime food restriction on causes, time, and predictors of death in dogs. J Am Vet Med Assoc 2005;226: 225–31.
10. Mattheeuws D, Rottiers R, Kaneko JJ, et al. Diabetes mellitus in dogs: relationship of obesity to glucose tolerance and insulin response. Am J Vet Res 1984;45: 98–103.
11. Klinkenberg H, Sallander MH, Hedhammar A. Feeding, exercise, and weight identified as risk factors in canine diabetes mellitus. J Nutr 2006;136:1985S–7S.
12. Lund EM, Armstrong PJ, Kirk CA, et al. Prevalence and risk factors for obesity in adult dogs from private US veterinary practices. Int J Appl Res Vet Med 2006;4: 177–86.
13. Scarlett JM, Donoghue S, Saidla J, et al. Overweight cats: prevalence and risk factors. Int J Obes Relat Metab Disord 1994;18(Suppl 1):S22–8.
14. Russell K, Sabin R, Holt S, et al. Influence of feeding regimen on body condition in the cat. J Small Anim Pract 2000;41:12–7.
15. Colliard L, Paragon BM, Lemuet B, et al. Prevalence and risk factors of obesity in an urban population of healthy cats. J Feline Med Surg 2009;11:135–40.
16. Courcier EA, O'Higgins R, Mellor DJ, et al. Prevalence and risk factors for feline obesity in a first opinion practice in Glasgow, Scotland. J Feline Med Surg 2010; 12:746–53.
17. Cave NJ, Allan FJ, Schokkenbroek SL, et al. A cross-sectional study to compare changes in the prevalence and risk factors for feline obesity between 1993 and 2007 in New Zealand. Prev Vet Med 2012;107:121–33.
18. Courcier EA, Mellor DJ, Pendlebury E, et al. An investigation into the epidemiology of feline obesity in Great Britain: results of a cross-sectional study of 47 companion animal practises. Vet Rec 2012;171:560.
19. Corbee RJ. Obesity in show cats. J Anim Physiol Anim Nutr (Berl) 2014;98: 1075–80.
20. Kronfeld DS, Donoghue S, Glickman LT. Body Condition and Energy Intakes of Dogs in a Referral Teaching Hospital. J Nutr 1991;121:S157–8.
21. McGreevy PD, Thomson PC, Pride C, et al. Prevalence of obesity in dogs examined by Australian veterinary practices and the risk factors involved. Vet Rec 2005;156:695–702.
22. Colliard L, Ancel J, Benet JJ, et al. Risk factors for obesity in dogs in France. J Nutr 2006;136:1951S–4S.

23. Weeth LP, Fascetti AJ, Kass PH, et al. Prevalence of obese dogs in a population of dogs with cancer. Am J Vet Res 2007;68:389–98.

24. Courcier EA, Thomson RM, Mellor DJ, et al. An epidemiological study of environmental factors associated with canine obesity. J Small Anim Pract 2010;51:362–7.

25. Corbee RJ. Obesity in show dogs. J Anim Physiol Anim Nutr (Berl) 2013;7: 904–10.

26. Mao J, Xia Z, Chen J, et al. Prevalence and risk factors for canine obesity surveyed in veterinary practices in Beijing, China. Prev Vet Med 2013;112:438–42.

27. White GA, Hobson-West P, Cobb K, et al. Canine obesity: is there a difference between veterinarian and owner perception? J Small Anim Pract 2011;52:622–6.

28. Holmes KL, Morris PJ, Abdulla Z, et al. Risk factors associated with excess body weight in dogs in the UK. J Anim Physiol Anim Nutr (Berl) 2007;91:166–7.

29. Courcier EA, Mellor DJ, Thomson RM, et al. A cross sectional study of the prevalence and risk factors for owner misperception of canine body shape in first opinion practice in Glasgow. Prev Vet Med 2011;102:66–74.

30. Allan FJ, Pfeiffer DU, Jones BR, et al. A cross-sectional study of risk factors for obesity in cats in New Zealand. Prev Vet Med 2000;46:183–96.

31. Levine ED, Erb HN, Schoenherr B, et al. Owner's perception of changes in behaviors associated with dieting in fat cats. J Vet Behav 2016;11:37–41.

32. Jeusette I, Greco D, Aquino F, et al. Effect of breed on body composition and comparison between various methods to estimate body composition in dogs. Res Vet Sci 2010;88:227–32.

33. Burger IH, Johnson JV. Dogs large and small: the allometry of energy requirements within a single species. J Nutr 1991;121:S18–21.

34. Serisier S, Weber M, Feugier A, et al. Maintenance energy requirements in miniature colony dogs. J Anim Physiol Anim Nutr (Berl) 2013;97(Suppl 1):60–7.

35. Kienzle E, Rainbird A. Maintenance energy requirement of dogs: what is the correct value for the calculation of metabolic body weight in dogs? J Nutr 1991;121: S39–40.

36. Bermingham EN, Thomas DG, Morris PJ, et al. Energy requirements of adult cats. Br J Nutr 2010;103:1083–93.

37. Bermingham EN, Thomas DG, Cave NJ, et al. Energy requirements of adult dogs: a meta-analysis. PLoS One 2014;9:e109681.

38. Raffan E, Smith SP, O'Rahilly S, et al. Development, factor structure and application of the Dog Obesity Risk and Appetite (DORA) questionnaire. PeerJ 2015;3: e1278.

39. Sallander M, Hagberg M, Hedhammar A, et al. Energy-intake and activity risk factors for owner-perceived obesity in a defined population of Swedish dogs. Prev Vet Med 2010;96:132–41.

40. Sloth C. Practical management of obesity in dogs and cats. J Small Anim Pract 1992;33:178–82.

41. Lefebvre SL, Yang M, Wang M, et al. Effect of age at gonadectomy on the probability of dogs becoming overweight. J Am Vet Med Assoc 2013;243:236–43.

42. Robertson ID. The influence of diet and other factors on owner-perceived obesity in privately owned cats from metropolitan Perth, Western Australia. Prev Vet Med 1999;40:75–85.

43. Fettman MJ, Stanton CA, Banks LL, et al. Effects of neutering on bodyweight, metabolic rate and glucose tolerance of domestic cats. Res Vet Sci 1997;62: 131–6.

44. Harper EJ, Stack DM, Watson TD, et al. Effects of feeding regimens on body-weight, composition and condition score in cats following ovariohysterectomy. J Small Anim Pract 2001;42:433–8.
45. Kanchuk ML, Backus RC, Calvert CC, et al. Weight gain in gonadectomized normal and lipoprotein lipase-deficient male domestic cats results from increased food intake and not decreased energy expenditure. J Nutr 2003;133:1866–74.
46. Alexander LG, Salt C, Thomas G, et al. Effects of neutering on food intake, body weight and body composition in growing female kittens. Br J Nutr 2011; 106(Suppl 1):S19–23.
47. Backus R. Plasma oestrogen changes in adult male cats after orchiectomy, body-weight gain and low-dosage oestradiol administration. Br J Nutr 2011; 106(Suppl 1):S15–8.
48. Belsito KR, Vester BM, Keel T, et al. Impact of ovariohysterectomy and food intake on body composition, physical activity, and adipose gene expression in cats. J Anim Sci 2009;87:594–602.
49. Scott KC, Levy JK, Gorman SP, et al. Body condition of feral cats and the effect of neutering. J Appl Anim Welf Sci 2002;5:203–13.
50. Backus RC, Cave NJ, Keisler DH. Gonadectomy and high dietary fat but not high dietary carbohydrate induce gains in body weight and fat of domestic cats. Br J Nutr 2007;98:641–50.
51. Nguyen PG, Dumon HJ, Siliart BS, et al. Effects of dietary fat and energy on body weight and composition after gonadectomy in cats. Am J Vet Res 2004;65: 1708–13.
52. Salmeri KR, Bloomberg MS, Scruggs SL, et al. Gonadectomy in immature dogs: effects on skeletal, physical, and behavioral development. J Am Vet Med Assoc 1991;198:1193–203.
53. Jeusette I, Detilleux J, Cuvelier C, et al. Ad libitum feeding following ovariectomy in female Beagle dogs: effect on maintenance energy requirement and on blood metabolites. J Anim Physiol Anim Nutr (Berl) 2004;88:117–21.
54. Serisier S, Feugier A, Venet C, et al. Faster growth rate in ad libitum-fed cats: a risk factor predicting the likelihood of becoming overweight during adulthood. J Nutr Sci 2013;2:e11.
55. Linder D, Mueller M. Pet obesity management: beyond nutrition. Vet Clin North Am Small Anim Pract 2014;44:789–806, vii.
56. Rowe E, Browne W, Casey R, et al. Risk factors identified for owner-reported feline obesity at around one year of age: dry diet and indoor lifestyle. Prev Vet Med 2015;121:273–81.
57. Hill RC. Challenges in measuring energy expenditure in companion animals: a clinician's perspective. J Nutr 2006;136:1967S–72S.
58. Handl S, Danninger-Dobrovits C, Iben C. Do feeding instructions on commercial dog foods promote obesity? In: Szymeczko R, Iben C, Burlikowska K, et al, editors. Proceedings of the 16th Congress of the European Society of Veterinary and Comparative Nutrition. Bydgoszcz (Poland): Multikop Sp. Z; 2012. p. 33.
59. Hervera M, Baucells MD, Torre C, et al. Prediction of digestible energy value of extruded dog food: comparison of methods. J Anim Physiol Anim Nutr (Berl) 2008;92:253–9.
60. National Research Council Ad Hoc Committee on Dog and Cat Nutrition. Energy. In: Nutrient requirements of dogs and cats. Washington, DC: National Academies Press; 2006. p. 28–48.
61. Bland IM, Guthrie-Jones A, Taylor RD, et al. Dog obesity: owner attitudes and behaviour. Prev Vet Med 2009;92:333–40.

62. Robertson ID. The association of exercise, diet and other factors with owner-perceived obesity in privately owned dogs from metropolitan Perth, WA. Prev Vet Med 2003;58:75–83.

63. Kienzle E, Bergler R, Mandernach A. A comparison of the feeding behavior and the human-animal relationship in owners of normal and obese dogs. J Nutr 1998; 128:2779S–82S.

64. German AJ, Holden SL, Gernon LJ, et al. Do feeding practices of obese dogs, before weight loss, affect the success of weight management? Br J Nutr 2011; 106(Suppl 1):S97–100.

65. Warren BS, Wakshlag JJ, Maley M, et al. Use of pedometers to measure the relationship of dog walking to body condition score in obese and non-obese dogs. Br J Nutr 2011;106(Suppl 1):S85–9.

66. Degeling C, Burton L, McCormack GR. An investigation of the association between socio-demographic factors, dog-exercise requirements, and the amount of walking dogs receive. Can J Vet Res 2012;76:235–40.

67. Suarez L, Pena C, Carreton E, et al. Preferences of owners of overweight dogs when buying commercial pet food. J Anim Physiol Anim Nutr (Berl) 2012;96: 655–9.

68. Nijland ML, Stam F, Seidell JC. Overweight in dogs, but not in cats, is related to overweight in their owners. Public Health Nutr 2010;13:102–6.

Development of Obesity
Mechanisms and Physiology

Robert Backus, MS, DVM, PhD, Allison Wara, DVM*

KEYWORDS

- Food intake control • Adiposity • Food reward • Satiation • Neutering • Exercise
- Metabolic rate • Physical activity

KEY POINTS

- Although body condition and adiposity seem regulated in adult animals, they likely reflect a net sum of influences on food intake and energy expenditure.
- Dietary manipulations that affect a satiation modality are not likely to have lasting effects on energy balance.
- Diets that are varied, highly palatable, and high in fat favor mismatching of energy expenditure with energy intake.
- Food intake control is determined by neuronal inputs of central and peripheral origin; however, physical activity is alterable and changes in total energy expenditure can induce and exacerbate the obese phenotype.

CONSTANCY OF BODY WEIGHT

It has long been observed that mature healthy animals when given free access to a nutritionally adequate diet typically maintain their body weight with little change over time. This attribute is a result of a robust physiologic mechanism. After adult animals are force-fed to an extent that they gain weight, with time, they lose weight if allowed ad libitum consumption. In these animals, transient reduction in food intake restores body weight to the initial condition. Conversely, if adult animals are deprived of food, body weight is lost until free access to food is restored. Body weight in this case is regained as food intake is increased and energy expenditure reduced. Unfortunately, body weight seems well defended even in animals that are overweight. In cases of obesity, the mechanism that stabilizes body weight becomes an impediment to treatments intended to restore a healthy body condition.

Disclosure Statement: The authors have nothing to disclose.
Department of Veterinary Medicine and Surgery, University of Missouri College of Veterinary Medicine, 900 East Campus Drive, Columbia, MO 65211, USA
* Corresponding author.
E-mail address: waraa@missouri.edu

Fat mass is the greatest of body constituents affected in maintenance of stable body weight. With long-term changes in food availability, change in body fat accounts for 90% of resulting body weight change. In times of food excess or deprivation, the amount of fat stored as triacylglycerol within cells of adipose varies and accounts most for the mass of adipose. The number and size of adipocytes increases with accretion of triacylglycerol, whereas when body fat is lost, adipocyte size decreases while adipocyte number is little affected.

The physiologic mechanism that stabilizes body weight and apparently defends a constant proportion body fat body is complex and incompletely understood. Over the long-term, when animals are in a state of body weight maintenance, energy intake matches energy expenditure. This energy balance may not be perturbed even when diets widely different in nutrient proportions and energy densities are consumed. On a day-to-day basis, the amount and type of food ingested varies, as does energy expenditure in physical activity and thermoregulation. Stabilizing environmental conditions and food presence does not eliminate daily variation in amount of energy consumed by animals. Food intake of humans with unrestricted access to a variety of foods may oscillate by an average of about 25% from day to day.[1] As daily food intake varies, compensatory energy expenditure generally follows, increasing and decreasing in proportion to food excess and deprivation, respectively. Hence, the mechanism that regulates body weight is necessarily complex and requires conditional weighting and integration of many cues and signals about food that are of internal and external origin.

FOOD INTAKE CONTROL

It is intuitive and true that control of food intake is a key component of the mechanism that regulates body weight. Food intake is a simple "on" and "off" act during which a "meal" is consumed. The frequency of meals in a day and the duration and amount of food consumed during a meal changes with food availability, experience, and environmental conditions. Animals eat many meals of differing sizes within a day when they are given free access to food, as is observed in dogs and cats presented with diets that maintain their palatability throughout a day (**Fig. 1**). Although the act of food intake

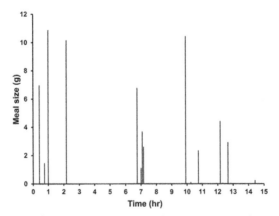

Fig. 1. Typical variation of meal size and periods of apparent satiety determined for an adult neutered male cat of stable body weight that is habituated to free access to a commercial dry feline diet during overnight (15 hour) periods. (*Courtesy of* Robert Backus, University of Missouri College of Veterinary Medicine, Columbia, MO.)

is simple, the elements responsible for its control are not simple. Food intake is a conditioned behavior compelled by motivations either to initiate or terminate a meal.[2] The motivations associated with food intake are determined by inputs of many neural circuits, which themselves are influenced by a myriad of signals of central and peripheral origin. Perceptions ascribed to motivations to eat and not to eat are hunger and satiety, respectively. Hunger influences when and how much to eat. With ingestion of food, hunger diminishes as a result of feedback. A feeling of fullness or satiation develops as eating continues so that eventually eating is terminated and a state of satiety is in effect. Eating should not resume until satiety or the feeling of being full wanes, and hunger again waxes.

SATIATION FACTORS

Inputs that affect the motivations to initiate or terminate food intake are diverse in kind.[3] Of these are signals that derive from sensed characteristics of food and from physiologic responses to food. Appearance, odor, and taste are among sensed characteristics that affect motivation to initiate food intake. Although important, they are characteristics that do not inform of energy value of food and their potency for affecting motivation to eat depends on prior experience. With food ingestion, stretch and chemoreceptors in the proximal gastrointestinal tract are activated. The signals that arise from these receptors provide satiation feedback but do not directly inform of the energy value of food. The signals influence meal size and duration but their potency for meal termination depends on prior experience. Later postingestive signals begin to provide information about the energy value of food and additionally serve as satiation feedback affecting meal termination. Glucose derived from food may be in the bloodstream within minutes of meal initiation. During this time the pattern of gut hormone secretion changes (eg, increased insulin, decreased glucagon) and so promotes a net uptake of nutrients by tissues. Input during the late ingestive phase may be satiating and contribute to signaling of meal termination. Meals end well before all nutrients of food are absorbed and their energy value is sensed in tissues that metabolize and store them. In animals given a diet of uniform and constant composition, early postingestive input seems relied on as a surrogate indicator of meal energy content. During the absorptive period and thereafter, the energy value of ingested food is presumed sensed. The means of sensing is unknown but it may relate to changes in rate of transfer, metabolism, and storage of nutrients. Additionally, depending on its kind, input of this postingestive phase may be integrated with other input resulting in decreasing satiety, increasing hunger, and initiation of food intake.

ADIPOSITY FACTORS

Other and especially important of inputs affecting food intake are those classified as adiposity signals. The presence of this kind of signaling was long suspected but only recently evinced. Adiposity signals are consistent with the so-called "lipostatic" theory, a hypothesis formulated in the early 1950s to explain body weight stability and its relationship with the amount of body fat an animal maintains.[4] The lipostatic theory postulates an internal mechanism that measures amount of body fat and in turn acts to adjust food intake in accord with the amount of energy needed to maintain a set-point in body fat. Although evidence for set-point in body fat mass is lacking, signals that indicate amount of body fat to neural circuits in the brain are demonstrated. A most clearly agreed on adiposity signal is plasma concentration of a protein called leptin, which is a name derived from the Greek word for thin.[5] Adipocytes secrete leptin into plasma in response to glucose and insulin and in proportion to their size, which is determined largely by their triacylglycerol load. Leptin concentration in plasma rises in proportion to body fat mass in many species, including dogs and cats.[6,7] Although a protein, leptin crosses the blood-brain barrier and once in the brain, it is a ligand to specific receptors on cells of many neural circuits. As circulating leptin rises, either as a result of gain in body fat or intravenous infusion, food intake is observed to decrease while energy expenditure increases. In this way, leptin in plasma is conceived to serve as an adiposity signal that feeds back to affect food intake and energy balance.

Insulin concentration in plasma is also considered by some investigators to be an adiposity signal.[8] Although insulin is a protein principally secreted by pancreatic endocrine cells and not adipose, concentrations of insulin are observed in many animals, including dogs and cats, to rise in plasma with increasing body fat. A feedback role for insulin is supported by several observations. Among these are that insulin crosses the blood-brain barrier, insulin is a ligand to receptors on neural circuits affecting food intake, and intracranial insulin infusions at physiologic doses reduce food intake.[8,9] An average rising circulating insulin concentration occurs with increasing adiposity because of resistance to the action of insulin for disposal of its nutrient secrectogogues, principally glucose and additionally amino acids, perhaps especially so for cats.[10] Other findings are not supportive of insulin as an adiposity signal. For example, in obese compared with lean states, food intake may be increased while plasma insulin concentration is high. However, for this case, obesity may be a consequence of resistance to action of insulin on food intake. Research in dogs indicates such insulin resistance could result from diminished transport of peripheral insulin to the brain.[11] Of worthy note here is that many cats once obese do not have extraordinarily great food intakes but they do have abnormally high plasma insulin concentrations.[12] High plasma insulin in obesity could be a braking signal functionally preventing further undesired gain in adiposity from continued overeating.

COGNITIVE FACTORS

Integration of inputs that affect control of food intake was once thought to occur in discrete centers of the brain. The current prevailing conception is that the decision to eat or not eat derives from activity of one complex brain circuit. The circuit receives signals from a great number and diversity of inputs that are interpreted and weighted against learning, experience, and environmental condition. This model of food intake control in part is favored because it accounts for cognition and stress effects, both of which are important to understanding causes and effective treatments of obesity. With this model, adiposity is not regulated to a set-point; it is rather believed to be a result of the net sum of influences on food intake and energy expenditure.[9]

Liking and wanting of a food or a characteristic of a food may develop beyond the energy value of a food. For this reason, adiposity is hypothesized to depend to some extent on the "reward" of pleasure and/or satisfaction that may be derived from food. This construct of food intake control postulates that the reward received varies with conditioning and the food presented. The risk of overeating and increased adiposity occur if the reward value is high. Food reward increases with the novelty and intake of highly palatable food. Brain circuits mediating the reward value of food have been identified during the past few decades. Unfortunately for prevention and treatment of obesity, they seem to be similar if not identical to those mediating the reward value of addictive drugs.[13] The food reward circuits include regions of the midbrain, limbic system, and cerebral cortex and involve dopaminergic and opioidergic neuron transmission. A role for reward circuits in food intake control is supported in findings of neural connections with brain regions integrating satiation, adiposity, and nutrient sensing that affect food intake.

Environment may also affect food intake control beyond homeostatic requirement for maintenance of energy balance. Environmental conditions may introduce cognitive stress, which for dogs and cats might be threatening situations, or lacking social interactions, or housing that is suboptimal for their temperament. Chronic cognitive stress most typically leads to reduced food intake and loss in body weight. However, studies of rodents under stress of this type and correlative human research reveals that food intake may be increased when food of high palatability is made available.[14] If prolonged, the increased food intake is followed by gain in body fat. The underling mechanism of such effects of stress is speculative. Chronic stress produces a sustained rise in circulating cortisol though stimulation of components of the hypothalamic-pituitary-adrenal axis. Cortisol is suggested to affect food intake control by attenuating adiposity signaling and enhancing food reward. Because food reward may dampen response to stressors, some comfort may be attained in stressful circumstances by consuming highly palatable food. Gain in body fat may be further promoted by cortisol through its inhibition of lipolysis in adipose and stimulation of proliferation and differentiation of adipocytes.

DIETARY MACRONUTRIENT AND FOOD INTAKE CONTROL

The energy that food provides is principally contained in the macronutrient classes of protein, fat, and carbohydrate. Of the macronutrients, dietary fat seems most promoting of undesired weight gain in dogs and cats. A few explanations for this effect of fat have been offered. Although dietary fat is much more energy dense than protein and carbohydrate, dietary fat may be less inhibiting of food intake in part because of its food reward potency. Aside from this, the energy in fat seems less effective at inhibiting food intake than energy from carbohydrate and protein. This discordance may be a result of a lower metabolic impact of fat compared with protein and carbohydrate. With excess energy intake, dietary protein and carbohydrate is preferentially oxidized, inhibiting fat oxidation. Even small amounts of dietary carbohydrate and to lesser degree dietary protein (except perhaps in cats) evoke insulin secretion. Elevation of circulating insulin inhibits lipolysis and release of fatty acids from adipose. Also with elevation in insulin, dietary lipids are sequestered in adipose from being oxidized. When in abundance, all macronutrients are somewhat stored in tissues, but among the macronutrients, an animal's capacity for fat storage is much greater and the energy cost for storage of fat is much lower.

MALADAPTIVE CHANGES

Of relevance to development of obesity in dogs and cats are several factors that may favor storage of body fat. The previously mentioned effect of cortisol that is elevated in chronic stress increases the number of adipocytes available for storage of fat. Increasing adipocyte number intuitively promotes accretion of body fat, but also it indirectly affects food intake control through diminished adiposity signaling. Leptin secretion by adipocytes rises exponentially as intracellular triacylglycerol increases.[5] Hence, for a given mass of body fat, increasing adipocyte number distributes stored triacylglycerol over more cells and reduces leptin secretion by these smaller cells. This phenomenon of adipocyte hyperplasia is relevant to understanding proclivity for regain of body fat in animals once obese. A ratchet-effect of adipocyte number occurs with cycles of weight gain and subsequent weight loss. Adipocyte hyperplasia is also relevant to justifying prevention of development of an undesired amount of adipose in young animals. Energy provision during development is well known to affect eventual adiposity in adulthood.[15] A life-long proclivity for obesity may be programmed in an overweight young animal. At birth, adipose is scarcely found in dogs and cats; but soon thereafter, its mass increases, and it increases in parallel with a growth spurt of the brain, where circuits of food intake control are maturing (**Fig. 2**).[16,17]

Dogs and cats are commonly neutered for behavioral reasons and for control of their populations. Although justifiable, an unfortunate consequence of neutering is increased risk for unwanted weight gain.[18] The weight gain of neutering principally reflects an expansion of adipose that is not driven by a change in the physiology of adipose. Lipoprotein lipase is a reputed gatekeeper of fat entry into adipose, yet cats that are naturally devoid of lipoprotein lipase become overweight when they are neutered.[19] The increased triacylglycerol store in the adipose of these neutered cats develops in parallel with their overeating. Neutering is observed to variably affect food intake and energy expenditure. For cats that are offered food for ad libitum consumption, a significant increase in food intake occurs within days of neutering. Detectable reduced energy expenditure may follow neutering. The lowering of energy expenditure in female cats may be substantial enough that maintenance of preneutering energy intake is too great to prevent gain in body weight.[20]

The neutering effect on food intake seems reflective of withdrawal of the gonad steroid hormones, estradiol and testosterone. Circulating estradiol concentration in males is similar to or greater than that of females except during estrus.[21,22] During estrus, estradiol concentrations greatly increase and seem to mediate a transient reduction in food intake in females. Metabolic conversion from testosterone is likely the principal source of estrogen in males. Administration of estradiol in physiologic concentrations to neutered cats restores food intake toward that of the preneuter state and prevents increased food intake and weight gain that follows neutering. The mechanism of action for the anorexic effect of estrogen is not completely understood. Estrogen seems to enhance the potency of satiation signals so that meal size is increased when its influence is withdrawn (**Fig. 3**).

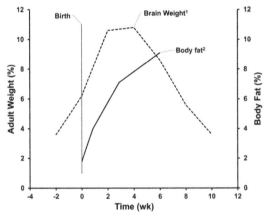

Fig. 2. Timing of expansions of brain and adipose mass relative to one another during the early perinatal period of cats. Superscripts of plot labels indicate sources of observations. (*Data from* Smith B, Jansen G. Brain development in the feline. Nutr Rep Int 1977;16:487–95; and Widdowson E. Food, growth and development in the suckling period. In: Graham-Jones O, editor. Canine and Feline Nutritional Requirements. Oxford: Pergamon Press; 1965. p. 9–17.)

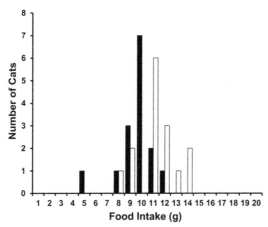

Fig. 3. Size of meals of male adult cats that are sexually intact (n = 8, *black bar*) and neutered (n = 8, *white bar*) when food was presented following overnight food withholding. The cats were habituated to a daily 4-hour interval of unrestricted presentation of a dry commercial feline diet. Body weights were not significantly different between the neutered and intact cats under this feeding paradigm. (*Data from* Backus R, Kanchuk M, Rogers Q. Elevation of plasma cholecystokinin concentration following a meal is increased by gonadectomy in male cats. J Anim Physiol Anim Nutr (Berl) 2006;90:152–8.)

With respect to energy balance, neutering may place dogs and cats at greater risk for overconsumption of energy, especially when dietary fat is high. In response to overconsumption, neutering may compromise the ability of some animals to compensate energy imbalance with increased energy expenditure. This is because energy expenditure may be reduced with neutering, which is more clearly demonstrated for cats than dogs.

ENERGY EXPENDITURE AND PHYSICAL ACTIVITY

Energy expenditure and physical activity are essential factors to consider in the pathogenesis of obesity. These two entities, however, are not equal and thus care must be taken to differentiate them. In humans, total energy expenditure (TEE) is classically defined as the sum of internal heat production (basal metabolic rate and dietary thermogenesis) plus external work (physical activity) (**Box 1**).[23]

Overall, dietary thermogenesis contributes to approximately 10% of TEE in dogs and in humans.[24] Studies evaluating the thermal effect of food on cats are lacking

---

Box 1
Energy expenditure and physical activity

TEE = internal heat production (basal metabolic rate + dietary thermogenesis) + external work

Basal metabolic rate refers to the energy required to maintain homeostasis in a postabsorptive state and depends on such factors as body weight, body composition, age, and reproductive status.[24] Dietary thermogenesis is an increase in internal heat production from the ingestion, digestion, absorption, and assimilation of nutrients, as well as activation of the autonomic nervous system.[24] Autonomic nervous system involvement has been shown in dogs during meal anticipation when catecholamines are released into circulation in response to the smell of food.[25]

but the contribution to TEE is thought to be similar. Basal metabolic rate and physical activity are highly variable and differ widely between individuals; therefore, the proportion of energy that these components contribute to TEE is inconstant.

Physical activity, however, can be defined as movement produced by skeletal muscle contraction that results in an increase in energy expenditure.[26] Physical activity can increase an individual's proportion of fat-free mass, which can influence overall body condition. In human patients, physical activity has been shown to prevent fat accretion and maintain or augment overall fat-free mass[27] compared with sedentary individuals. A recent study[28] conducted on client-owned overweight or obese dogs demonstrated that individuals involved in a physical training program showed improved preservation of lean body mass (as measured by dual-energy x-ray absorptiometry) during weight loss, compared with control dogs receiving caloric restriction only.

Although the pathophysiologic mechanisms responsible for the development of obesity are complex and multifactorial, a decrease in spontaneous physical activity and/or a decrease in energy expenditure are important contributing factors. Thus, when considering the development of the obese phenotype, one must also consider the individual components that can impact physical activity and energy expenditure.

FACTORS THAT CAN INFLUENCE PHYSICAL ACTIVITY AND/OR ENERGY EXPENDITURE

Independent of body weight, body composition can largely impact an individual's energy expenditure, specifically via the percentage of lean body mass in relation to fat mass. Adipose tissue is metabolically less active than lean body tissue and therefore metabolic rates are lower in obese individuals compared with lean (**Box 2**).[24]

Social interaction is another modifiable lifestyle factor that has been shown to impact physical activity. Hubrecht and colleagues[30] demonstrated that dogs housed in solitary quarters were inactive up to 85% of the time, whereas those that were group-housed and granted opportunities for social interaction were inactive for only 54% to 62% of the time.

Although physical activity is typically considered voluntary, there is growing evidence to support the theory that it can also be modulated by biologic parameters. Sex hormones, such as estrogen and testosterone, contribute greatly to the regulation of physiologic factors and thus play an important role in patterns of physical activity across various species including humans. Much of the work in this field has been documented in rodent models with an extensive and well-established history.

In male and female rats, it has been long-observed that castration and ovariectomy significantly decreases physical activity because of alterations in sex hormones.[29,31] Furthermore, in aromatase-deficient mice that cannot synthesize endogenous estrogens, increased adiposity resulted, in part, from reduced physical activity, not hyperphagia or decreased resting energy expenditure.[32]

Although administration of either testosterone or estradiol to male castrated rats resulted in an increase in spontaneous activity, estradiol elicited a greater response,

---

Box 2
Measuring energy expenditure

In a group of Beagles, energy expenditure was measured as 130 ± 6 kcal/kg body weight$^{0.75}$ for dogs in normal body condition with 25% body fat using a doubly labeled water technique.[29] When these dogs were permissively overfed such that they accumulated excessive body fat (38%), energy expenditure decreased to 107 ± 7 kcal/kg body weight$^{0.75}$.

presumably because of the aromatization of testosterone into estrogen that precedes its biologic action.[33] Moreover, implantation of ovarian tissue into altered male and female rats restored activity to physiologic levels[34] and supplementation with 17β-estradiol to ovariectomized mice recovered preneutering activity patterns.[35]

There is strong evidence pointing to the hypothesis that estrogenic activation of the estrogen-α receptor pathway is the physiologic mechanism through which spontaneous activity is increased or augmented.[36] Subsequently, sex differences in physical activity patterns of rodents are also observed, with females exhibiting significantly increased daily activity levels compared with males.[37] Recent work has further evaluated this association by demonstrating an increase in the speed, distance, and duration of wheel-running by female mice compared with males.[38]

Despite the number of studies investigating the effects of sex hormones on physical activity in rodents, the data available on dogs and cats are limited. One study[39] quantitatively measured physical activity in group-housed cats using collar-mounted accelerometers before and after ovariohysterectomy. They reported a 52% overall decrease in physical activity in the spayed group compared with intact control animals.

In another study,[19] energy expenditure was measured in colony cats using a double-label water technique to determine whether the pattern of weight gain following gonadectomy was a result of increased energy intake or decreased energy expenditure. Despite a rapid increase in food intake 2 days following gonadectomy, metabolic rates before and after alteration were overall unchanged. Although this is a field of great interest, it is clear that further research is required for validation of the effects of sex hormones on physical activity in companion animals.

Leptin is another hormone that has been well-recognized to have a significant impact on energy balance in various species. This adipocyte-derived cytokine hormone targets receptors in the arcuate nucleus of the hypothalamus to regulate satiety and maintain energy homeostasis.[40] The DNA sequence encoding for leptin was first detected in rodent models on the obese (ob) gene and mutations in this gene are associated with hyperphagia, reduced energy expenditure, and severe obesity.[41] To investigate the in vivo physiologic effects of leptin in mice, one study[42] continuously monitored energy expenditure, oxygen consumption, and respiratory quotient via open-circuit calorimetry. Obese mice (ob/ob), which have been characterized as having reduced activity levels compared with control animals, showed an increase in energy expenditure following intraperitoneal administration of leptin.

In addition to energy expenditure, the effects of leptin on physical activity have also been documented. Choi and colleagues[43] found that when leptin was administered intracerebroventricularly, the hormone significantly stimulated spontaneous physical activity in rats, in addition to suppressing food intake and weight gain.

Conversely, leptin resistance, a syndrome characterized by a failure of increased concentrations of endogenous leptin to modulate increased appetite and decreased energy expenditure in the face of overnutrition, is also thought to play a potential role in the pathogenesis of obesity.[44] Although there is a paucity of data to substantiate the presence of leptin resistance in dogs or cats, it is conceivable that this mechanism may also be a causative factor of obesity in companion animals.

SUMMARY

Long-term balance of energy expenditure with energy intake is precisely controlled via complex and incompletely understood mechanisms such that body weight and adiposity seem regulated and defended, even in animals that sustain an overweight body condition. Dietary and environmental factors including dietary fat and palatability, inactive and stressful lifestyle, and neutering are relevant to promotion of the overweight body condition.

REFERENCES

1. Flatt J. Issues and misconceptions about obesity. Obesity (Silver Spring) 2011; 19:676–86.
2. Blundell J, Gibbons C, Caudwell P, et al. Appetite control and energy balance: impact of exercise. Obes Rev 2015;16(Suppl 1):67–76.
3. Koopmans H. Experimental studies on the control of food intake. In: Bray GA, Bouchard C, editors. Handbook of obesity, etiology and pathophysiology. 2nd edition. New York: Marcel Dekker; 2004. p. 373–425.
4. Kennedy G. The role of depot fat in the hypothalamic control of food intake in the rat. Proc R Soc Lond B Biol Sci 1953;140:578–96.
5. Houseknecht KL, Baile CA, Matteri RL, et al. The biology of leptin: a review. J Anim Sci 1998;76:1405–20.
6. Backus R, Havel P, Gingerich R, et al. Relationship between serum leptin immunoreactivity and body fat mass as estimated by use of a novel gas-phase Fourier transform infrared spectroscopy deuterium dilution method in cats. Am J Vet Res 2000;61:796–801.
7. Ishioka K, Soliman M, Sagawa M, et al. Experimental and clinical studies on plasma leptin in obese dogs. J Vet Med Sci 2002;64:349–53.
8. Porte D Jr, Woods S. Regulation of food intake and body weight in insulin. Diabetologia 1981;20(Suppl):274–80.
9. Woods S, Begg D. Regulation of the motivation to eat. Curr Top Behav Neurosci 2015. [Epub ahead of print].
10. Curry D, Morris J, Rogers Q, et al. Dynamics of insulin and glucagon secretion by the isolated perfused cat pancreas. Comp Biochem Physiol A Comp Physiol 1982;72:333–8.
11. Kaiyala K, Prigeon R, Kahn S, et al. Obesity induced by a high-fat diet is associated with reduced brain insulin transport in dogs. Diabetes 2000;49:1525–33.
12. Hoenig M, Thomaseth K, Waldron M, et al. Insulin sensitivity, fat distribution, and adipocytokine response to different diets in lean and obese cats before and after weight loss. Am J Physiol Regul Integr Comp Physiol 2007;292:R227–34.
13. Figlewicz D, Sipols A. Energy regulatory signals and food reward. Pharmacol Biochem Behav 2010;97:15–24.
14. Adam T, Epel E. Stress, eating and the reward system. Physiol Behav 2007;91: 449–58.
15. Spencer S. Early life programming of obesity: the impact of the perinatal environment on the development of obesity and metabolic dysfunction in the offspring. Curr Diabetes Rev 2012;8:55–68.
16. Widdowson E. Food, growth and development in the suckling period. In: Graham-Jones O, editor. Canine and feline nutritional requirements. Oxford (United Kingdom): Pergamon Press; 1965. p. 9–17.
17. Smith B, Jansen G. Brain development in the feline. J Nutr Rep Int 1977;16: 487–95.
18. McGreevy P, Thomson P, Pride C, et al. Prevalence of obesity in dogs examined by Australian veterinary practices and the risk factors involved. Vet Rec 2005; 156:695–702.

19. Kanchuk M, Backus R, Calvert C, et al. Weight gain in gonadectomized normal and lipoprotein lipase-deficient male domestic cats results from increased food intake and not decreased energy expenditure. J Nutr 2003;133:1866–74.

20. Root M, Johnston S, Olson P. Effect of prepuberal and postpuberal gonadectomy on heat production measured by indirect calorimetry in male and female domestic cats. Am J Vet Res 1996;57:371–4.

21. Backus R. Plasma oestrogen changes in adult male cats after orchiectomy, body-weight gain and low-dosage oestradiol administration. Br J Nutr 2011;106(Suppl 1):S15–8.

22. de Gier J, Buijtels J, Albers-Wolthers C, et al. Effects of gonadotropin-releasing hormone administration on the pituitary-gonadal axis in male and female dogs before and after gonadectomy. Theriogenology 2012;77:967–78.

23. Arciero PJ, Nindl BC. Obesity. In: LeMura LM, von Duvillard SP, editors. Clinical exercise physiology: application and physiological principles. Philadelphia: Lippincott Williams & Wilkins; 2004. p. 303–18.

24. National Research Council of the National Academies. Energy. In: Nutrient requirements of dogs and cats. Washington, DC: The National Academies Press; 2006. p. 28–48.

25. Diamond P, Brondel L, Leblanc J. Palatability and postprandial thermogenesis in dogs. Am J Physiol 1985;248:E75–9.

26. Heath G. Behavioral approaches to physical activity promotion. In: Ehrman J, Gordon P, Visich P, et al, editors. Clinical exercise physiology. 2nd edition. Champaign (IL): Human Kinetics; 2009. p. 17–30.

27. Kyle U, Gremion G, Genton L, et al. Physical activity and fat-free and fat mass by bioelectrical impedance in 3853 adults. Med Sci Sports Exerc 2001;33(4):576–84.

28. Vitger A, Stallknecht B, Nielsen D, et al. Integration of a physical training program in a weight loss plan for overweight pet dogs. J Am Vet Med Assoc 2016;248(2):174–82.

29. Hoskins R. The effect of castration on voluntary activity. Am J Physiol 1925;72:324–30.

30. Hubrecht R, Seppel J, Poole T. Correlates of pen size and housing conditions on the behavior of kenneled dogs. Appl Anim Behav Sci 1992;34:365–83.

31. Slonaker J. The effect of pubescence, oestruation and menopause on the voluntary activity in the albino rat. Am J Physiol 1924;68:294–315.

32. Jones M, Thorburn A, Britt K, et al. Aromatase-deficient (ArKO) mice accumulate excess adipose tissue. J Steroid Biochem Mol Biol 2001;79:3–9.

33. Roy E, Wade G. Role of estrogens in androgen-induced spontaneous activity in male rats. J Comp Physiol Psychol 1975;89:573–9.

34. Lightfoot J. Sex hormones' regulation of rodent physical activity: a review. Int J Biol Sci 2008;4(3):126–32.

35. Gorzek J, Hendrickson K, Forstner J, et al. Estradiol and tamoxifen reverse ovariectomy-induced physical inactivity in mice. Med Sci Sports Exerc 2007;39:248–57.

36. Garey J, Morgan M, Frohlich J, et al. Effects of the phytoestrogen coumestrol on locomotor and fear-related behaviors in female mice. Horm Behav 2001;40:65–76.

37. Bronstein P, Wolkoff F, Levine M. Sex-related differences in rats' open-field activity. Behav Biol 1975;13:133–8.

38. Lightfoot J, Turner M, Pomp D, et al. Quantitative trait loci for physical activity traits in mice. Physiol Genomics 2008;32(3):401–8.

39. Belsito K, Vester B, Keel T, et al. Impact of ovariohysterectomy and food intake on body composition, physical activity, and adipose gene expression in cats. J Anim Sci 2009;87:594–602.

40. Klok M, Jakobsdottir S, Drent M. The role of leptin and ghrelin in the regulation of food intake and body weight in humans: a review. Obes Rev 2007;8(1):21–34.

41. Zhang Y, Proenca R, Maffei M, et al. Positional cloning of the mouse obese gene and its human homologue. Nature 1994;372:425–32.

42. Hwa J, Fawzi A, Graziano M, et al. Leptin increases energy expenditure and selectively promotes fat metabolism in ob/ob mice. Am J Physiol 1997;272(4 Pt 2):R1204–9.

43. Choi Y, Li C, Hartzell D, et al. ICV leptin effects on spontaneous physical activity and feeding behavior in rats. Behav Brain Res 2008;188(1):100–8.

44. Scarpace P, Zhang Y. Leptin resistance: a predisposing factor for diet-induced obesity. Am J Physiol Regul Integr Comp Physiol 2009;296:493–500.

Current Topics in Canine and Feline Obesity

Beth Hamper, DVM, PhD

KEYWORDS

- Canine • Feline • Obesity • Nutrition • Neuter

KEY POINTS

- The onset of obesity leads to alterations in thousands of genes, including peroxisome proliferator-activated receptor γ, sterol regulatory element-binding protein-1, adiponectin, glucose transporter type 4, and uncoupling proteins.
- Obesity in most instances is a polygenic disorder.
- Single mutations in FTO (fat mass and obesity-associated protein), MC4R (melanocortin-4 receptor), and PPARG (peroxisome proliferator-activated receptor γ) are associated with marked obesity in humans, but their function significance in dogs and cats is unknown.
- Gut microflora diversity is reduced in obese dogs compared with lean dogs.
- Gene transcription modifications may preclude clinical signs, which may be a useful diagnostic tool in the management and treatment of obesity.

INTRODUCTION

Obesity is now the most common nutritional disorder in dogs and cats.[1] Numerous factors can predispose an animal to obesity, including genetics, neutering, decreased activity level, gut microbiota, and high fat/high energy diets. Research investigating causes and treatment are currently primarily limited to rodent or human models, with comparatively fewer data in dogs and cats. This article reviews current research in canine and feline obesity with comparisons to human and rodent studies where applicable.

GENETICS

Obesity is generally a polygenic disorder, with relevant genes interacting with environmental factors to contribute to obesity.[2]

Rodents

The ob/ob (obese)[3] and db/db (diabetic) mice[4] are examples of single gene mutations that result in obesity. Genetic studies have found that the ob/ob mouse has a single

Disclosure Statement: The author has nothing to disclose.
Hamper Veterinary Nutritional Consulting, 9160 Crestview Drive, Indianapolis, IN 46240, USA
E-mail address: hamp0003@umn.edu

base pair deletion for the protein hormone leptin, whereas the db/db mouse has a mutation in leptin's receptor.

Humans

Human studies show that 40% to 70% of interindividual variation in obesity risk and body mass index is genetic.[5] The phenotypic effects of most genetic polymorphisms are small with few single mutations causing marked obesity. These cases are rare (1%–6% of obese humans) and typically involve mutations in the fat mass and obesity-associated protein (FTO), melanocortin-4 receptor (MC4R), or peroxisome proliferator-activated receptor γ (PPARG) genes.[6–8] These genes play important roles because of their effects on energy balance, appetite, and satiety.

The MC4R gene, encoding a transmembrane G-protein–coupled receptor expressed mainly in the hypothalamus, is implicated as a susceptibility gene in human diabetes mellitus and obesity, as it plays an important role in regulating energy balance and appetite.[9–11] In a situation of positive energy balance, MC4R is stimulated by α–melanocyte–stimulating hormone (α-MSH), causing satiety. In starvation, the activity of MC4R is inhibited by its inverse antagonist, agouti-related protein, causing hunger.[11] Mutations in MC4R are the most common single genetic cause of human obesity (up to 6% of cases).[7]

Canine

The canine and feline genomes have been sequenced.[12,13] Canine MC4R, FTO and PPARG gene polymorphisms are identified, but their functional significance has not been determined. Single nucleotide polymorphisms (SNPs) of the MC4R gene have been identified in various groups of dogs, but no significant association has been found between these and canine obesity per se.[14,15] In beagle dogs, 2 single nucleotide polymorphisms in the MC4R gene were associated with increased body weight and were proposed as a genetic marker for selecting dog size.[16]

Feline

MC4R polymorphisms have been associated with diabetes mellitus in overweight domestic short-haired cats.[17] The feline MC4R polymorphisms were not related to increased susceptibility to obesity, but rather diminished glycemic control in the presence of insulin resistance. In young cats (less than 1 year old), a yet unknown genetic factor has been proposed in their development of obesity.[18]

ADIPOSE TISSUE AND ADIPOKINES

White adipose tissue is the major storage form of excess dietary energy. Initially, thought of as an inert tissue, it has been increasingly recognized as an important endocrine organ that secretes a variety of substances including steroid hormones, growth factors, proteins, cytokines, and regulators of lipid metabolism.[19] Taken together, these substances are named *adipokines* and are defined as biologically active substances produced in adipose tissue that act via autocrine, paracrine, or endocrine mechanisms. Proinflammatory adipokines include leptin, tumor necrosis factor α (TNF-α), interleukin-6 (IL-6), and resistin. A few others, particularly adiponectin, exert anti-inflammatory effects and may protect against metabolic disturbances.[20] (See Melissa Clark and Margarethe Hoenig's article, "Metabolic Effects of Obesity and Its Interaction with Endocrine Diseases," in this issue.)

NUTRACEUTICALS

Several nutraceuticals, including soy isoflavones, carnitine, and the combination of diacylglycerols (DAGs) and low glycemic index starch (LGIS) have been evaluated for use in companion animal weight loss diets.

Canine

Dogs given soy isoflavones supplements have shown a greater loss of fat and increased likelihood of achieving target body fat compared with controls fed a similar unsupplemented calorie-restricted diet.[21] To the author's knowledge, there have been no peer-reviewed studies evaluating carnitine for weight loss in dogs.

DAGs are lipids that contain 2 fatty acid chains esterified to glycerol compared with triacylglycerols, which have 3 fatty acids. The fatty acids from DAG have been reported to enhance fat oxidization and are metabolized differently.[22] Dogs given DAG supplements lost weight and had lower serum triglyceride concentrations than triacylglyceride-supplemented controls, whereas control dogs maintained body weight.[23] LGIS (ie, amylose) is hydrolyzed more slowly than other types of starch, thereby providing a slower, more consistent, source of glucose. It is expected that this starch would stimulate less insulin release compared with starches with higher glycemic index values (HGIS, ie, amylopectin). Because insulin stimulates lipogenesis and inhibits lipolysis, it is possible that more weight loss may be achieved with longer-term ingestion of LGIS-containing foods than HGIS-containing food.[24] Overweight dogs fed a diet containing LGIS lost more weight than those fed an HGIS-based diet.[22] Based on this finding, dogs fed LGIS and DAG may be able to control weight and maintain serum lipid levels without reduction in caloric intake.

Feline

Male and female cats fed isoflavones (genistein) supplements after neutering had less body fat and more lean muscle tissue than unsupplemented control cats.[25]

Carnitine is produced endogenously from the amino acids, lysine and methionine, and is required for transport of lipids into the mitochondrial matrix for oxidation. Because there is endogenous synthesis of carnitine, supplementation is likely to be of greatest benefit when protein intake is limited. Carnitine supplementation for weight loss has shown mixed results.[21,26–29] A significant increase in body weight loss in cats carnitine supplements compared with a control group was reported,[28,30] and Shoveller and colleagues[29] reported that with carnitine supplementation, overweight cats had greater energy expenditure and motivation to play, whereas there was no effect in lean cats. (See Deborah E. Linder and Valerie J. Parker's article, "Dietary Aspects of Weight Management in Cats and Dogs," in this issue, for further information on integrating nutraceutical therapy into a nutritional plan for weight loss.)

"Omics"

Advances in molecular biology have opened new areas of research including omic studies. The neologism *omics* refers to a field of biology aimed at collective characterization and quantification of biological molecules. For example, *genomics* refers to the study of the genome and gene expression in an organism. **Table 1** lists the various different fields of omics studies. Despite progress, limited information and molecular tools are available for studying mechanisms of obesity in dogs and cats using an omics approach. Studies specific to dogs and cats, and factors and mechanisms contributing to companion animal obesity will be reviewed. Common gene expression responses to body weight gain and obesity are shown in **Fig. 1.**

Table 1
Various omics definitions

Genomics	Study of the Genome and its Function in an Organism
Transciptomics	Study of the transcriptions including mRNA, tRNA, rRNA; their structure and function
Proteomics	Study of the entire compliment of proteins produced, including modifications made
Lipidomics	Study of the networks and pathways of lipids in an organism
Metabolomics	Study of small molecule metabolite profiles associated with cellular processes
Nutrigenomics	Study of the effects of foods and food constituents on the genome, proteome, and metabolome

Canine Studies

Canine white adipose tissue expresses many protein adipokines associated with inflammation including adiponectin, leptin, IL-6, haptoglobin, monocyte chemoattractant protein-1, TNF-α, and nerve growth factor (NGF).[31,32] NGF, central to the development and maintenance of sympathetic innervation, is also an inflammatory response protein in adipose tissue.[33] Treatment of the differentiated canine adipocytes with lipopolysaccharide (LPS) resulted in a dramatic increase in NGF mRNA and NGF; treatment with TNF-α caused an increase in NGF mRNA and NGF, whereas

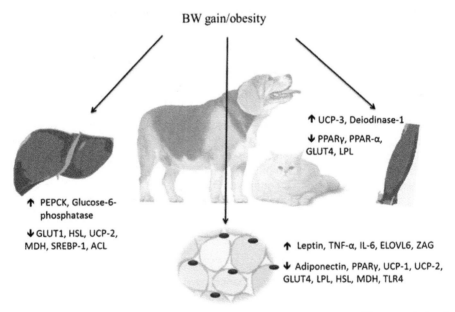

Fig. 1. Effects of pet obesity or body weight gain on gene expression of hepatic, skeletal muscle, and adipose tissues. ELOVL6, elongation of long-chain fatty acids family member 6; GLUT, glucose transporter; MDH, malate dehydrogenase; PEPCK, phosphoenolpyruvate carboxykinase; PPAR, peroxisome proliferator-activated receptor; TLR, toll-like receptor; ZAG, zinc-2 α glycoprotein. (*From* de Godoy MR, Swanson KS. Companion Animals Symposium: nutrigenomics: using gene expression and molecular biology data to understand pet obesity. J Anim Sci 2013;91(6):2954; with permission.)

IL-6 treatment had little effect.[34] Treatment of these cells with dexamethasone decreased both NGF mRNA and NGF protein release, and the PPARG agonist, rosiglitazone, reduced NGF secretion.[34] These results show that canine adipocytes express and secrete key adipokines, and are highly reactive to inflammatory mediators and signals.

During the development of obesity, adipose tissue undergoes major expansion and remodeling. In one study of laboratory dogs, global gene expression profiles of adipose tissue in dogs fed a high-fat diet, during the transition from a lean to obese phenotype, were analyzed. Ad libitum feeding increased body weight, body fat mass, adipocyte size, and leptin levels.[35] The onset of obesity also altered expression of 1665 genes in adipose tissue. Several related functional gene classes including transcription, transport, carbohydrate and lipid metabolism, signaling, cell cycle, differentiation and growth, and RNA processing were affected.[35] Genes related to oxidative stress were upregulated during early weight gain and may relate to increases in adipocyte cell size. Client-owned obese dogs have also been examined. Increases in concentrations of TNF-α, C-reactive protein, insulin, and insulin/glucose have been observed.[36] Further, weight loss caused decreases in these same variables, which improved insulin sensitivity and diminished inflammatory processes.[36]

Several studies evaluated PPARG expression in dogs fed high-fat diets, comparing lean and obese states. PPARG, a member of the nuclear receptor superfamily, is highly enriched in adipocytes and macrophages. It is involved in adipocyte differentiation, regulates fatty acid storage and glucose metabolism, and increases expression of uncoupling proteins (UCPs). PPARG modulates expression of genes for glucose and lipid metabolism, including glucose transporter type 4 (GLUT4), lipoprotein lipase (LPL), leptin, and adiponectin. Uncoupling proteins are mitochondrial carrier proteins that catalyze a regulated proton leak across the inner mitochondrial membrane, diverting free energy from adenosine triphosphate (ATP) synthesis to the production of heat.[37] UCPs modulate cold- and diet-induced heat production, contributing to adaptive changes in energy expenditure. UCPs contribute to regulation of whole-body energy balance, and their dysfunction may contribute to obesity.[38] Dogs fed a high-fat diet to achieve obesity and insulin resistance showed decreases in visceral fat PPARG mRNA expression (from 100%–23%) and UCP1 mRNA expression (from 100%–24%) compared with measurements made at baseline (normal weight).[39] The effects of obesity on expression of PPARG-targeted genes in lean and obese dogs has also been examined in a similar study. In the similarly induced obese and insulin resistance dogs,[40] plasma leptin and triglycerides increased, whereas plasma adiponectin decreased. Furthermore, transcription of mRNA for adiponectin, PPARG, GLUT4, and LPL were all decreased,[40] suggesting that development of insulin resistance with associated reduced GLUT4 mRNA transcription and translocation of GLUT4 protein may be the result of reduced transcription of PPARG.

Effects of a high-fat diet on mRNA transcription of LPL, PPARG, hormone-sensitive lipase (HSL), and genes involved in gluconeogenesis (glucose 6-phosphatase and phosphoenolpyruvate carboxylase) have also been investigated.[41] Compared with control-fed dogs, those fed a high-fat diet had an increased ratio of visceral to subcutaneous mRNA transcription of both LPL and PPARG and greater expression of sterol regulatory element-binding protein-1 (SREBP-1). SREBP-1 is involved in cholesterol, free fatty acid, and triglyceride synthesis.[42] HSL was also increased in visceral fat, indicating upregulation of lipolysis. In addition, glucose-6-phosphatase and phosphoenolpyruvate carboxykinase increased, consistent with enhanced gluconeogenesis. Liver triglyceride content was 45% higher, and insulin receptor binding was 50% lower, in high fat–fed dogs versus controls. Expression of genes promoting lipid accumulation and lipolysis in visceral fat, as well as increases in hepatic rate-limiting gluconeogenic enzymes are consistent with the portal theory, which infers that high rates of lipolysis from the large intra-abdominal adipose depot cause excess free fatty acid flux to the liver via the portal vein. This, in turn, leads to hepatic insulin resistance and triglyceride accumulation in the hepatocytes. This same group later found that obese dogs fed a high-fat diet led to enlarged adipocytes primarily in the visceral fat depot.[43] Visceral adipocytes larger than 75 μm were considered to be good predictors of whole-body and hepatic insulin resistance, whereas size of adipocytes in subcutaneous adipose tissue was not.[43]

Only a few studies have approached nutrigenomics in obese dogs. Effects of feeding short-chain fructooligosaccharides on insulin resistance and adipose tissue metabolism in obese dogs were evaluated[44] in research dogs fed to achieve obesity and insulin resistance. Supplementation with short-chain fructooligosaccharides decreased insulin resistance, which was potentially explained by increased expression of UCP2 and carnitine palmitoyltransferase-1, which regulates fatty acid oxidation.

Green tea supplementation in obese insulin-resistant dogs[45] improved insulin sensitivity by 60%. The supplement did not result in weight loss or reduced fat mass but did decrease plasma triglycerides by 50% and increased expression of PPARG, LPL, GLUT4, and adiponectin in visceral and subcutaneous adipose tissue.

Feline Studies

Cats can digest and metabolize high levels of dietary fat.[46] Several lipases regulate lipid depot size and function. LPL facilitates the tissue uptake of free fatty acids.[47] HSL is an intracellular enzyme responsible for hydrolysis of triglycerides and release of free fatty acids and glycerol into the circulation.[48] Compared with lean controls, obese cats had reduced plasma LPL, decreased LPL mRNA in subcutaneous fat, and increased LPL and HSL mRNA in skeletal muscle.[49] Muscle TNF-α was not different between groups, but obese cats had higher adipocyte TNF-α concentrations than lean cats. The lower LPL activity and mRNA expression in fat and the higher LPL and HSL mRNA expression in muscle in obese cats suggest redistribution of fatty acids from fat to muscle tissue where they can be deposited or used for energy in times of need. TNF-α may be an important regulator of this repartitioning through suppression of adipocyte LPL.[49]

Positive energy balance can chronically activate SREBP-1, resulting in increased expression of the lipogenic enzymes ATP citrate lyase (ACL) and fatty acid synthase (FAS). SREBP-1 is a transcription factor involved with lipogenesis and adipocyte development, whereas ACL is a cytosolic enzyme that catalyzes the synthesis of acetyl-CoA for de novo synthesis of fatty acids. FAS catalyzes fatty acid synthesis and is transcriptionally regulated by SREBP-1 in response to insulin and food intake. In experimentally induced overweight cats,[50] FAS and SREBP-1 expression were significantly increased in omental adipose tissue whereas ACL, FAS, and SREBP-1c expressions were significantly decreased in subcutaneous adipose tissues compared with healthy controls. These results suggest that omental adipose tissue seems to foster, whereas subcutaneous adipose and liver tissues seem to defer, lipid storage based on differences in SREBP-1 mRNA expression.[50]

In cats that were food restricted for 12 weeks after spaying and then fed ad libitum for 12 weeks, adipose tissue LPL, HSL, and adiponectin mRNA decreased and adipose IL-6 was increased at week 24 compared with baseline. It is also reported in cats that gene expression of adipose adiponectin, HSL, and UCP decreases, whereas GLUT4 expression increases with ovariohysterectomy-associated weight gain. In skeletal muscle, GLUT1, HSL and UCP gene expression decreases. These 2 studies found that ovariohysterectomy may establish a new setpoint characterized by specific physiologic changes.

Thyroid hormones exert many of their effects on energy metabolism by affecting gene transcription. Triiodothyronine (T3) increases basal metabolic rate and has been proposed to regulate UCP.[51] UCP2 predominates in adipose, whereas UCP3 predominates in muscle.[52] Both increase under conditions of increased energy expenditure, such as fever, hyperthyroidism, high leptin concentrations, and cold exposure.[52] Regulation of UCP2 is mediated by PPARG.[52] T3 administration[53] increased thermogenesis without changing UCP expression in lean and obese cats, showing that T3 does regulate thermogenesis in cats but not through uncoupling proteins.

GUT MICROBIOTA

Typical changes in gut microbiota associated with obesity in humans are characterized by reduced bacterial diversity and reduced representation of the phylum Bacteroidetes, and enrichment in carbohydrate and lipid-utilizing genes in the microbiome overall.[54] Several mechanisms implicate the microbiome in obesity development and propagation. These include utilization of energy from nondigestible carbohydrates, manipulation of host gene functions, and exacerbation of inflammation.[55]

Diet is clearly a determinant of obesity through excess energy intake and is also a primary determinant of gastrointestinal microbiota composition. Studies in animals and humans found that dietary modification results in rapid alterations to microbiota composition.[56] Several studies found mechanisms for low-grade systemic inflammation associated with high-fat diets.[57,58] Increases in dietary fat alter LPS absorption with increased intestinal absorption into the lymph. High-fat diets have been found to chronically increase plasma LPS concentrations 2- to 3-fold. A high-fat diet also increases proportions of LPS-containing bacteria in the gut.[58]

Rodents

A causal relationship between alterations in gut microbiota and body weight has been found in rodents. Recipient germ-free mice receiving gut microbiota from obese versus lean donors differed markedly in adiposity. Within 2 weeks, animals that received the microbiota from obese donors gained significantly more body fat and extracted more calories from food than mice receiving microbiota from lean donors.[59]

Canine

Two studies examined the microbiome in obese dogs.[60,61] Evaluation of the fecal microbiome of lean and obese dogs (pets and research animals)[60] showed dominance of the phylum Firmicutes (mean abundance >90%), whereas Actinobacteria, Fusobacteria, Proteobacteria and Bacteroidetes were also identified. The mean abundance of Actinobacteria was greater in obese dogs. At the genus level, *Roseburia* (0.66% vs 0.21%) was more abundant in obese dogs, and the order Clostridiales was increased under ad libitum feeding in research dogs. Similar to humans, canine intestinal microbiota was highly diverse with a high degree of interindividual variation. When fecal microbiomes of obese research dogs and lean controls were compared in another study,[61] the phylum Firmicutes (85.2%) was the most dominant group, with Actinobacteria (7.94%) more abundant than Bacteroidetes (2.34%) in the lean dogs, whereas the predominant phylum in the obese group was Proteobacteria. The order Clostridiales was markedly more abundant in the lean group compared with the obese group, and the proportion of Pseudomonadales was markedly higher in the obese group compared with the lean group. Similar to microbiome in humans, the diversity of microbial communities was lower in the obese group.[61]

Feline

Clinical studies examining dysbiosis in feline inflammatory disease exist,[62,63] but further work is needed to understand the role of gut microbiota in the physiologic, pathologic, and underlying mechanisms of obesity in cats.

SUMMARY

Obesity is a significant health problem for humans and companion animals. Genetics, diet, and environmental factors all play a role in its development. The application of new research tools is needed to further understand the underlying mechanisms and causality of obesity development in dogs and cats so that realistic interventions can be made for improving animal (and human) health.

REFERENCES

1. German A. The growing problem of obesity in dogs and cats. In: 2006 World Congress Proceedings 31st World Small Animal Association Congress, 12th European Congress FECAVA, & 14th Czech Small Animal Veterinary Association Congress. Prague, Czech Republic, October 11-14, 2006. p. 377–78.
2. Speakman J, Hambly C, Mitchell S, et al. The contribution of animal models to the study of obesity. Lab Anim 2008;42(4):413–32.
3. Zhang Y, Proenca R, Maffei M, et al. Positional cloning of the mouse obese gene and its human homolog. Nature 1994;372(6505):425–32.
4. Lee GH, Proenca R, Montez JM, et al. Abnormal splicing of the leptin receptor in diabetic mice. Nature 1996;379(6566):632–5.
5. Day FR, Loos RJF. Developments in obesity genetics in the era of genome-wide association studies. J Nutrigenet Nutrigenomics 2011;4(4):222–38.
6. Razquin C, Marti A, Alfredo Martinez J. Evidences on three relevant obesogenes: MC4R, FTO and PPAR gamma. Approaches for personalized nutrition. Mol Nutr Food Res 2011;55(1):136–49.
7. Santini F, Maffei M, Pelosini C, et al. Melanocortin-4 receptor mutations in obesity. In: Makowski GS, editor. Advances in clinical chemistry, vol. 48. San Diego (CA): Elsevier Academic Press Inc; 2009. p. 95–109.
8. Wardle J, Carnell S, Haworth CMA, et al. Obesity associated genetic variation in FTO is associated with diminished satiety. J Clin Endocrinol Metab 2008;93(9): 3640–3.
9. Xi B, Takeuchi F, Chandak GR, et al. Common polymorphism near the MC4R gene is associated with type 2 diabetes: data from a meta-analysis of 123,373 individuals. Diabetologia 2012;55(10):2660–6.
10. Lindgren CM, Loos RJ, Li S, et al. Association studies involving over 90,000 samples demonstrate that common variants near to MC4R influence fat mass, weight and risk of obesity. Diabetes 2008;57:A485–6.
11. Cone RD. Anatomy and regulation of the central melanocortin system. Nat Neurosci 2005;8(5):571–8.
12. Lindblad-Toh K, Wade CM, Mikkelsen TS, et al. Genome sequence, comparative analysis and haplotype structure of the domestic dog. Nature 2005;438(7069): 803–19.
13. Pontius JU, Mullikin JC, Smith DR, et al. Initial sequence and comparative analysis of the cat genome. Genome Res 2007;17(11):1675–89.

14. Skorczyk A, Stachowiak M, Szczerbal I, et al. Polymorphism and chromosomal location of the MC4R (melanocortin-4 receptor) gene in the dog and red fox. Gene 2007;392:247–52.

15. van den Berg L, van den Berg SM, Martens EECP, et al. Analysis of variation in the melanocortin-4 receptor gene (mc4r) in golden retriever dogs. Anim Genet 2010;41(5):557.

16. RuiXia Z, YiBo Z, Peng D. The SNPs of melanocortin 4 receptor (MC4R) associated with body weight in Beagle dogs. Exp Anim 2014;63(1):73–8.

17. Forcada Y, Holder A, Church DB, et al. A polymorphism in the melanocortin 4 receptor gene (MC4R:c.92C > T) is associated with diabetes mellitus in overweight domestic shorthaired cats. J Vet Intern Med 2014;28(2):458–64.

18. Haring T, Haase B, Zini E, et al. Overweight and impaired insulin sensitivity present in growing cats. J Anim Physiol Anim Nutr 2013;97(5):813–9.

19. Sethi JK, Vidal-Puig AJ. Thematic review series: Adipocyte biology - Adipose tissue function and plasticity orchestrate nutritional adaptation. J Lipid Res 2007;48(6):1253–62.

20. Pan W, Kastin AJ. Adipokines and the blood-brain barrier. Peptides 2007;28(6):1317–30.

21. Pan Y. Use of soy isoflavones for weight management in spayed/neutered dogs. FASEB J 2006;20(5):A854–5.

22. Mitsuhashi Y, Nagaoka D, Ishioka K, et al. Postprandial lipid-related metabolites are altered in dogs fed dietary diacylglycerol and low glycemic index starch during weight loss. J Nutr 2010;140(10):1815–23.

23. Umeda T, Bauer JE, Otsuji K. Weight loss effect of dietary diacylglycerol in obese dogs. J Anim Physiol Anim Nutr 2006;90(5–6):208–15.

24. Brand-Miller JC, Holt SHA, Pawlak DB, et al. Glycemic index and obesity. Am J Clin Nutr 2002;76(1):281S–5S.

25. Cave NJ, Backus RC, Marks SL, et al. Oestradiol, but not genistein, inhibits the rise in food intake following gonadectomy in cats, but genistein is associated with an increase in lean body mass. J Anim Physiol Anim Nutr 2007;91(9–10):400–10.

26. Brandsch C, Eder K. Effect of L-carnitine on weight loss and body composition of rats fed a hypocaloric diet. Ann Nutr Metab 2002;46(5):205–10.

27. Aoki MS, Almeida A, Navarro F, et al. Carnitine supplementation fails to maximize fat mass loss induced by endurance training in rats. Ann Nutr Metab 2004;48(2):90–4.

28. Center SA, Harte J, Watrous D, et al. The clinical and metabolic effects of rapid weight loss in obese pet cats and the influence of supplemental oral L-carnitine. J Vet Intern Med 2000;14(6):598–608.

29. Shoveller AK, Minikhiem DL, Carnagey K, et al. Low level of supplemental dietary l-camitine increases energy expenditure in overweight, but not lean, cats fed a moderate energy density diet to maintain body weight. Intern J Appl Res Vet Med 2014;12(1):33–43.

30. Center SA, Warner KL, Randolph JE, et al. Influence of dietary supplementation with L-carnitine on metabolic rate, fatty acid oxidation, body condition, and weight loss in overweight cats. Am J Vet Res 2012;73(7):1002–15.

31. Wood IS, German AJ, Hunter L, et al. Adipokine gene expression in dog adipose tissues and dog white adipocytes differentiated in primary culture. Horm Metab Res 2005;37(8):474–81.

32. Ryan VH, German AJ, Wood IS, et al. Adipokine expression and secretion by canine adipocytes: stimulation of inflammatory adipokine production by LPS and TNFalpha. Pflugers Arch 2010;460(3):603–16.

33. Trayhurn P, Wood IS. Adipokines: inflammation and the pleiotropic role of white adipose tissue. Br J Nutr 2004;92(3):347–55.
34. Ryan VH, German AJ, Wood IS, et al. NGF gene expression and secretion by canine adipocytes in primary culture: upregulation by the inflammatory mediators LPS and TNF alpha. Horm Metab Res 2008;40(12):861–8.
35. Grant RW, Vester Boler BM, Ridge TK, et al. Adipose tissue transcriptome changes during obesity development in female dogs. Physiol Genomics 2011; 43(6):295–307.
36. German AJ, Hervera A, Hunter L, et al. Improvement in insulin resistance and reduction in plasma inflammatory adipokines after weight loss in obese dogs. Domest Anim Endocrinol 2009;37(4):214–26.
37. Boss O, Hagen T, Lowell BB. Uncoupling proteins 2 and 3-Potential regulators of mitochondrial energy metabolism. Diabetes 2000;49(2):143–56.
38. Enerback S, Jacobsson A, Simpson EM, et al. Mice lacking mitochondrial uncoupling protein are cold-sensitive but not obese. Nature 1997;387(6628):90–4.
39. Leray V, Gayet C, Martin L, et al. Modulation of uncoupling protein 1 and peroxisome proliferator-activated receptor gamma expression in adipose tissue in obese insulin-resistant dogs. J Nutr 2004;134(8):2154S–7S.
40. Gayet C, Leray V, Saito M, et al. The effects of obesity-associated insulin resistance on mRNA expression of peroxisome proliferator-activated receptor-gamma target genes, in dogs. Br J Nutr 2007;98(3):497–503.
41. Kabir M, Catalano KJ, Ananthnarayan S, et al. Molecular evidence supporting the portal theory: a causative link between visceral adiposity and hepatic insulin resistance. Am J Physiol Endocrinol Metab 2005;288(2):E454–61.
42. Jackson SM, Ericsson J, Metherall JE, et al. Role for sterol regulatory element binding protein in the regulation of farnesyl diphosphate synthase and in the control of cellular levels of cholesterol and triglyceride: evidence from sterol regulation-defective cells. J Lipid Res 1996;37(8):1712–21.
43. Kabir M, Stefanovski D, Hsu IR, et al. Large size cells in the visceral adipose depot predict insulin resistance in the canine model. Obesity (Silver Spring) 2011;19(11):2121–9.
44. Respondek F, Swanson KS, Belsiro KR, et al. Short-chain fructooligosaccharides influence insulin sensitivity and gene expression of fat tissue in obese dogs. J Nutr 2008;138(9):1712–8.
45. Serisier S, Leray V, Poudroux W, et al. Effects of green tea on insulin sensitivity, lipid profile and expression of PPAR alpha and PPAR gamma and their target genes in obese dogs. Br J Nutr 2008;99(6):1208–16.
46. Butterwick RF, Salt C, Watson TDG. Effects of increases in dietary fat intake on plasma lipid and lipoprotein cholesterol concentrations and associated enzyme activities in cats. Am J Vet Res 2012;73(1):62–7.
47. Mead JR, Irvine SA, Ramji DP. Lipoprotein lipase: structure, function, regulation, and role in disease. J Mol Med 2002;80(12):753–69.
48. Kraemer FB, Shen WJ. Hormone-sensitive lipase: control of intracellular tri-(di-)acylglycerol and cholesteryl ester hydrolysis. J Lipid Res 2002; 43(10):1585–94.
49. Hoenig M, McGoldrick JB, deBeer M, et al. Activity and tissue-specific expression of lipases and tumor-necrosis factor alpha in lean and obese cats. Domest Anim Endocrinol 2006;30(4):333–44.
50. Lee P, Mori A, Takemitsu H, et al. Lipogenic gene expression in abdominal adipose and liver tissues of diet-induced overweight cats. Vet J 2011;190(2): e150–3.

51. Gong DW, He YF, Karas M, et al. Uncoupling protein-3 is a mediator of thermogenesis regulated by thyroid hormone, beta 3-adrenergic agonists, and leptin. J Biol Chem 1997;272(39):24129–32.
52. Lanni A, Moreno M, Lombardi A, et al. Thyroid hormone and uncoupling proteins. FEBS Lett 2003;543(1–3):5–10.
53. Hoenig M, Caffall Z, Ferguson DC. Triiodothyronine differentially regulates key metabolic factors in lean and obese cats. Domest Anim Endocrinol 2008;34(3): 229–37.
54. Turnbaugh PJ, Hamady M, Yatsunenko T, et al. A core gut microbiome in obese and lean twins. Nature 2009;457(7228):480–4.
55. Graham C, Mullen A, Whelan K. Obesity and the gastrointestinal microbiota: a review of associations and mechanisms. Nutr Rev 2015;73(6):376–85.
56. David LA, Maurice CF, Carmody RN, et al. Diet rapidly and reproducibly alters the human gut microbiome. Nature 2014;505(7484):559–63.
57. Cani PD, Neyrinck AM, Fava F, et al. Selective increases of bifidobacteria in gut microflora improve high-fat-diet-induced diabetes in mice through a mechanism associated with endotoxaemia. Diabetologia 2007;50(11):2374–83.
58. Cani PD, Amar J, Iglesias MA, et al. Metabolic endotoxemia initiates obesity and insulin resistance. Diabetes 2007;56(7):1761–72.
59. Backhed F, Ding H, Wang T, et al. The gut microbiota as an environmental factor that regulates fat storage. Proc Natl Acad Sci U S A 2004;101(44):15718–23.
60. Handl S, German AJ, Holden SL, et al. Faecal microbiota in lean and obese dogs. FEMS Microbiol Ecol 2013;84(2):332–43.
61. Park H-J, Lee S-E, Kim H-B, et al. Association of obesity with serum leptin, adiponectin, and serotonin and gut microflora in beagle dogs. J Vet Intern Med 2015; 29(1):43–50.
62. Inness VL, McCartney AL, Khoo C, et al. Molecular characterisation of the gut microflora of healthy and inflammatory bowel disease cats using fluorescence in situ hybridisation with special reference to Desulfovibrio spp. J Anim Physiol Anim Nutr 2007;91(1–2):48–53.
63. Janeczko S, Atwater D, Bogel E, et al. The relationship of mucosal bacteria to duodenal histopathology, cytokine mRNA, and clinical disease activity in cats with inflammatory bowel disease. Vet Microbiol 2008;128(1–2):178–93.

Metabolic Effects of Obesity and Its Interaction with Endocrine Diseases

Melissa Clark, DVM, PhD[a],*,
Margarethe Hoenig, DVM, PhD, Dr med vet[b]

KEYWORDS

- Obesity • Canine • Feline • Insulin resistance • Dyslipidemia • Diabetes
- Hepatic lipidosis • Adipocytokines

KEY POINTS

- Obesity in dogs and cats leads to numerous metabolic and endocrine abnormalities, including insulin resistance, altered adipokine secretion, blood lipid disorders, and ectopic fat accumulation.
- The effects of insulin resistance are initially limited by a compensatory increase in insulin secretion; if concurrent beta cell dysfunction develops, diabetes may ensue, particularly in cats.
- Altered lipid metabolism and hepatic triglyceride deposition may contribute to the predisposition of obese cats to hepatic lipidosis.
- Although the concept of a "metabolic syndrome" has been investigated in dogs and cats, no system currently exists to predict development of obesity-related metabolic complications.

INTRODUCTION

Obesity in pet dogs and cats is a significant problem in developed countries, and seems to be increasing in prevalence.[1] In dogs and cats, as in other species, accumulation of excess body fat has numerous adverse metabolic consequences. Adipose tissue, once thought to be an inert storage depot, has been recognized as an endocrine organ that actively participates in carbohydrate and lipid metabolism, energy regulation, and the inflammatory and coagulation cascades.[2] In the setting of overnutrition and obesity, control of these processes is altered; although this may not be immediately apparent clinically, altered glucose and lipid metabolism can ultimately

The authors have nothing to disclose.
[a] Department of Internal Medicine, The Animal Medical Center, 510 East 62nd Street, New York, NY 10065, USA; [b] Department of Veterinary Clinical Medicine, College of Veterinary Medicine, University of Illinois at Urbana-Champaign, 1008 West Hazelwood Drive, Urbana-Champaign, IL 61802, USA
* Corresponding author.
E-mail address: melissa.clark@amcny.org

predispose to diabetes mellitus (DM) and/or hepatic lipidosis (HL), and changes in energy metabolism may contribute to difficulty correcting obesity, particularly in cats. This article reviews the metabolic and endocrine changes known to occur with development of obesity in dogs and cats, and discusses their clinical significance.

NORMAL METABOLIC FUNCTION OF ADIPOSE TISSUE
Lipid Storage and Release

Mammalian white adipose tissue is specialized for the uptake, processing, and storage of circulating lipids. Lipids circulating as triglycerides (either dietary or endogenous) are hydrolyzed to yield glycerol and nonesterified fatty acids (NEFAs) on encountering the enzyme lipoprotein lipase on endothelial cells. These NEFAs are quickly taken up by fatty acid transporters on the surfaces of adipocytes, and most are re-esterified into triglycerides for intracellular storage. During times of energy deficit, triglycerides are hydrolyzed and NEFAs are released through the actions of intracellular lipases (eg, adipocyte triglyceride lipase, hormone-sensitive lipases).[3]

NEFAs may be taken up by other tissues such as muscle and liver to be used for energy or re-esterified for export or storage. Unlike adipose tissue, however, liver and muscle are not specialized for lipid storage, and accumulation of large amounts of intracellular triglyceride would be detrimental to normal cellular function. Therefore, in times of fuel surfeit or increased NEFA concentrations, uptake and sequestration of lipids by adipose tissue seems to act as a buffer protecting lean tissues from ectopic lipid deposition.

Endocrine Functions

Adipose tissue contains receptors for a wide variety of endocrine hormones, including insulin, glucagon, growth hormone, thyroid hormone, angiotensin, incretins, and glucocorticoids, as well as for catecholamines and cytokines such as interleukin (IL)-6 and tumor necrosis factor (TNF)-α.[2] Thus, it is able to respond to metabolic signals from other organ systems to help coordinate fuel storage and utilization. In turn, adipocytes themselves produce and release substances that participate in interorgan communication. These include the adipose-derived cytokines (or "adipokines"), adiponectin and leptin, along with proteins for lipid transport and components of the inflammatory and coagulation cascades. Adiponectin, produced exclusively by adipose tissue, has insulin-sensitizing and antiinflammatory properties, whereas leptin exerts central control of appetite and energy expenditure.[2]

The importance of adipose tissue in overall fuel and energy metabolism can be appreciated by observing the effect of adipose tissue depletion: laboratory mice that lack adipose tissue develop severe insulin resistance, diabetes, dyslipidemia, and ectopic lipid deposition, and similar metabolic derangements are observed in humans with lipoatrophy or lipodystrophy.[4,5]

Obesity, adipose tissue dysfunction, and the metabolic syndrome

Although a deficiency of adipose tissue is clearly detrimental from a metabolic standpoint, excess adipose tissue has equally deleterious consequences. In humans, the development of obesity is associated with a constellation of metabolic abnormalities that predispose to type 2 DM and cardiovascular disease. These abnormalities are collectively termed "the metabolic syndrome," and include central adiposity, evidence of insulin resistance, blood lipid disorders, and systemic hypertension.[6] In addition to DM and cardiovascular disease, nonalcoholic fatty liver disease (a chronic hepatopathy characterized by excessive lipid accumulation in the liver, with subsequent inflammation and hepatic dysfunction) and reproductive disorders (eg, polycystic ovarian syndrome) are considered potential sequelae of the metabolic syndrome in humans.[6,7]

The specific mechanisms by which nutrient or adipose tissue excess lead to metabolic dysregulation have not been clearly defined. However, this is an active area of study in human medicine, and potential mechanisms include:

- Cellular hypoxia resulting from adipocyte hypertrophy, which leads to oxidative stress, apoptosis, and an inflammatory response that negatively impacts fuel metabolism[8,9];
- Decreased adipocyte mitochondrial function, independent of cell size[10];
- Altered secretion of adipokines and other bioactive substances, including those involved in insulin sensitivity and inflammation[6]; and
- Abnormal fatty acid trafficking that results in increased delivery of lipids to lean tissue and intracellular accumulation of lipid intermediates (eg, fatty acyl coenzyme A, ceramides, and diacylglycerol) that interfere with insulin signaling.[11,12]

Therefore, at least in humans and rodents, it seems that increased fat mass results in a reduced ability of adipose tissue to perform its usual metabolic roles, beginning at a molecular level and culminating in systemic consequences. The effects of obesity on adipose tissue have been referred to as "adiposopathy" or "adipose tissue dysfunction" by some investigators (**Box 1**).[13,14]

Many of the same metabolic abnormalities noted in humans occur with canine and feline obesity, and attempts have been made to define an analogue to the metabolic syndrome in dogs.[15] However, in pets, there has been less correlation of obesity-induced metabolic abnormalities with long-term outcomes, and significant species differences exist. Specific metabolic changes known to occur with obesity in dogs and cats, and exploration of the concept of metabolic syndrome in dogs, are discussed in the following sections.

OBESITY, INSULIN RESISTANCE, AND HYPERINSULINEMIA

One of the most well-recognized changes that occurs with excess adiposity is insulin resistance, or a diminished cellular response to a given plasma insulin concentration. In healthy individuals, the binding of insulin to its cell surface receptors triggers a signaling cascade that promotes glucose uptake and glycogen formation in muscle, inhibits endogenous glucose production (EGP) in the liver, and increases glucose and lipid uptake and inhibits lipolysis in adipose tissue.[3,16] Insulin sensitivity and

---

Box 1
Adipose tissue dysfunction in obesity

- In humans and rodents, increased fat mass may result in "adiposopathy," or a reduced ability of adipose tissue to perform its usual metabolic roles.[13,14]
  - This begins on a molecular level and culminates in systemic consequences.

- Potential mechanisms for adipose tissue dysfunction in obesity include:
  - Cellular hypoxia subsequent to adipocyte hypertrophy
    - May lead to oxidative stress, apoptosis, and an inflammatory response that negatively impacts fuel metabolism[8,9];
  - Decreased adipocyte mitochondrial function[10];
  - Altered secretion of adipokines and other bioactive substances, including those involved in insulin sensitivity and inflammation[6];
  - Abnormal fatty acid trafficking and intracellular accumulation of lipid intermediates that interfere with insulin signaling.[11,12]

resistance are classically assessed by the euglycemic–hyperinsulinemic clamp (EHC), in which insulin is infused at a variable rate to keep blood glucose within a set of pre-determined parameters. The infusion rate necessary to accomplish this is an indicator of the response of peripheral tissues to insulin, that is, the less insulin necessary to control blood glucose, the more insulin-sensitive the individual.

In humans, a multiple-dose EHC with isotopic tracers (to determine the origin of circulating glucose and fatty acids) has shown that obesity leads to insulin resistance in all 3 major metabolic organs (adipose tissue, muscle, and the liver).[17] That is, in obese individuals, the responses to insulin in these organs are blunted, and higher concentrations of insulin are needed to keep plasma glucose and free fatty acid con-centrations within normal limits. During everyday conditions, these higher concentra-tions of insulin are supplied endogenously: plasma insulin concentrations in obese humans are 20% to 50% greater than in lean humans.[17,18] This response to insulin resistance occurs in obese rodents and other mammals and is referred to as compen-satory hyperinsulinemia.[18,19]

Although a multiple-dose tracer EHC has not been reported in dogs or cats, a single-dose EHC in cats has demonstrated a 30% decrease in insulin sensitivity with each 1-kg increase in body weight.[20] In addition, multiple investigators have shown decreased glucose clearance during intravenous glucose tolerance tests (IVGTT) in obese cats.[20–22] In the IVGTT, a bolus of glucose is administered to stimulate endogenous in-sulin release, and the declining plasma glucose concentration is measured over 2 to 3 hours afterward. Plasma insulin concentration is also measured, and values reflecting both glucose clearance and insulin sensitivity can be calculated from IVGTT data.

- In a longitudinal study of weight gain in cats, in which IVGTTs were performed after gain of 0%, 10%, 30%, 60%, and 100% over lean body weight, a 17% decrease in insulin sensitivity and a 15% decrease in insulin-independent glucose uptake were found per kilogram of weight gain. Additionally, there was a statistically significant increase in glucose area under the curve at 60% weight gain or greater.[23]
- In an earlier study, expression of the insulin-dependent glucose transporter GLUT-4 in both muscle and fat was found to be lower in obese than in lean cats,[24] suggesting a possible mechanism for decreased glucose uptake.

Insulin resistance has also been demonstrated in obese dogs using EHC,[25] and decreased glucose clearance in obese dogs, starting at gain of 40% over lean body weight, has been shown using IVGTT.[26] Additionally, both basal insulin concentrations and insulin area under the curve during IVGTT are increased in obese dogs and cats, as they are in other mammals.[26–30] In the aforementioned longitudinal studies of feline obesity, these changes were apparent with as little as 10% gain over lean body weight (**Fig. 1**).[23] Traditionally, compensatory hyperinsulinemia has been thought to result from an increase in beta cell mass[31,32]; however, decreased insulin clearance has been shown in obese, hyperinsulinemic dogs.[33]

Of note, pharmacologic doses of glucose used in IVGTT in dogs and cats do not reflect the routine concentrations to which pancreatic beta cells are subjected after a meal. Therefore, results should be interpreted with caution, especially with regard to application to daily glucose homeostasis and beta cell function.

GLUCOSE CONCENTRATIONS IN OBESITY

Despite peripheral insulin resistance, obese cats and dogs are able to maintain normal plasma glucose concentrations for extended periods of time. A cross-sectional study

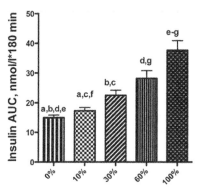

Fig. 1. Mean ± standard error area under the curve (AUC) for insulin concentrations during intravenous glucose tolerance testing in cats at 10%, 30%, 60%, and 100% gain over lean body weight. (*From* Hoenig M, Pach N, Thomaseth K, et al. Cats differ from other species in their cytokine and antioxidant enzyme response when developing obesity. Obesity (Silver Spring) 2013;21:E410; with permission.)

of 117 client-owned cats (normal weight, overweight, obese, and naïve or treated diabetic) found no difference in basal blood glucose or fructosamine concentrations between the overweight/obese and normal weight cats.[34] Other values on routine clinicopathologic assessment (complete blood count, serum biochemistry, total thyroxine [T4], and feline pancreatic lipase) also did not differ among these groups, with the exception of triglyceride concentrations, which were higher in overweight and obese than in normal cats. There was a distinct delineation between fructosamine values of overweight and obese cats and those of diabetic cats, without identification of an intermediate "prediabetic" state (eg, a gradation of glucose or fructosamine concentrations) in this cohort.

Another study investigated 24-hour plasma glucose concentrations in lean and long-term obese cats via continuous glucose monitoring and found no difference in blood glucose concentration between groups throughout the day.[35] Similarly, plasma glucose concentrations do not necessarily rise with obesity or decline with weight loss in dogs.[15,25,36]

For fasting plasma glucose to remain within normal limits despite a decreased ability to clear glucose from circulation, EGP by the liver must be controlled, because the liver is the major source of blood glucose during fasting. EGP has been shown to be lower in obese than in lean cats when normalized for body weight, possibly as a result of the suppressive effect of increased insulin concentrations on hepatic glucose production.[28] Thus far, no studies are available to characterize changes in hepatic glucose output with obesity in dogs.

PREDISPOSITION TO DIABETES MELLITUS

Obesity is a known risk factor for DM in humans and cats; obese cats are 2 to 4 times more likely to be diabetic than are cats of normal body condition.[37,38] Insulin resistance is thought to be involved in this predisposition, and it has been postulated that the increased secretory demand associated with obesity-induced insulin resistance eventually leads to depletion of pancreatic insulin stores and beta cell exhaustion.[39] However, the latter mechanism has been demonstrated primarily in situations of preexisting beta cell compromise (eg, Matsuda and asscociates[40]), and many obese cats and humans never develop DM, despite years of insulin resistance. There-fore, long-term peripheral insulin resistance is not a sole prerequisite for the progres-sion to a diabetic state, and concurrent beta cell functional compromise must be present.

Proposed mechanisms of obesity-related beta cell compromise include (1) interfer-ence by nutrient excess with insulin signaling in beta cells[39] (leading to loss of normal trophic feedback and beta cell apoptosis) and (2) increased pancreatic deposition of amyloid in humans and cats, consequent to hypersecretion of the amyloid precursor amylin in insulin-resistant states.[41] Amyloid fibrils are toxic to beta cells in vitro,[42,43] and pancreatic amyloid deposits are present in many diabetic cats and are associated with decreased beta cell mass.[44] However, they are also present in approximately 45% of older nondiabetic cats, although they are not as extensive as in diabetic cats.[45] Therefore, increased amylin secretion and amyloid deposition are not the sole determinants of beta cell failure in feline DM, although they may contribute by decreasing beta cell functional reserve.[44,46]

In support of the concept that both insulin resistance and beta cell function contribute to the onset of type 2 DM, the natural history of type 2 DM in a genetically predisposed human population involves (1) a period of peripheral insulin resistance with hyperinsulinemia and euglycemia, (2) a decline in beta cell function with impaired insulin secretory response to glucose and decreased glucose tolerance, and (3) further reduction in insulin secretion with loss of hepatic insulin sensitivity and loss of control of EGP.[47] A similar pattern, with initial loss of the first phase of insulin secretion during IVGTT and impaired glucose tolerance, and later a decrease in overall insulin concentrations, has been observed in partially pancreatectomized cats rendered insu-lin resistant by administration of growth hormone and dexamethasone.[22] In both pop-ulations, overt hyperglycemia occurred when insulin secretory reserve became inadequate to overcome preexisting insulin resistance. Thus, apart from any direct effect of obesity on the beta cell, obesity-induced insulin resistance may simply in-crease the likelihood of metabolic decompensation when other stresses on the beta cell (either genetic or environmental) are present. A summary of possible factors involved in progression from obesity-induced insulin resistance to diabetes in cats is illustrated in **Fig. 2**.

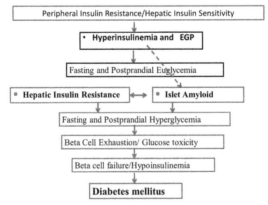

Fig. 2. Proposed sequence of events in progression from obesity-induced insulin resistance to diabetes mellitus in cats. EGP, endogenous glucose production. (*From* Hoenig M. Carbohydrate metabolism and pathogenesis of diabetes mellitus in dogs and cats. Prog Mol Biol Trans Sci 2014;121:403.)

The relationship between obesity and DM in dogs is less clear, because evidence of an autoimmune pathogenesis has been demonstrated in diabetic dogs[48] and early studies of diabetes in dogs suggested that most cases were associated with advanced beta cell failure.[49] However, a subset of diabetic dogs with obesity, insulin resistance, and high endogenous insulin secretion, but poor insulin secretory response to glucose, has been described.[49] Additionally, according to a study from a large chain of US veterinary hospitals, the prevalence of obesity and of DM in dogs has increased in a similar fashion over the past several years, suggesting that there is a connection between the two, and that reassessment of obesity as a risk factor for DM in dogs may be indicated.[1]

ADIPOKINE SECRETION IN OBESITY

One possible mechanism contributing to insulin resistance in obese animals and humans is altered secretion of adipocyte-derived cytokines. The most well-known of these cytokines are leptin and adiponectin, although numerous others (eg, resistin, retinol-binding protein 4, apelin, and nicotinamide phophoribosyltransferase) have been described.[6,50]

Leptin

Leptin was the first of the traditional adipokines to be identified, as the missing gene product in the obese, hyperphagic *ob/ob* mouse.[51] Its concentration is proportional to fat mass and decreases during fasting, prompting an increase in appetite (through reduced activation of receptors in the hypothalamic satiety center), a decrease in overall metabolic rate, upregulation of the hypothalamic–pituitary–adrenal axis, and downregulation of the hypothalamic–pituitary–thyroid and hypothalamic–pituitary–gonadal axes. These changes are reversed when food consumption resumes and leptin concentration increases. Thus, under normal physiologic circumstances, leptin acts to maintain energy homeostasis during fasting and refeeding. In addition, the structure of leptin is similar to that of IL-6, and it exhibits proinflammatory activity.[6]

In dogs and cats, as in other mammals, plasma leptin concentration increases with expansion of fat mass[20,52,53] and decreases with weight loss.[20,54] However, the higher leptin concentrations of obese humans and pets do not seem to suppress appetite, leading to a hypothesis of "leptin resistance" (possibly involving impaired leptin signaling or decreased transport through the blood-brain barrier) in obesity.[52,55] Additionally, increased leptin concentrations are not accompanied by a corresponding increase in energy expenditure in obese cats (see discussion below).

Adiponectin

Adiponectin is the most abundant gene product of adipose tissue, and circulates at relatively high concentrations (μg/mL) in plasma. It may be present as low-molecular-weight or high-molecular-weight (HMW) multimers; in humans, the HMW forms seem to be most active biologically.[50] Binding of adiponectin to its receptors in skeletal muscle and liver increases beta-oxidation of fatty acids, reduces intracellular triglyceride content and improves insulin sensitivity.[2] Adiponectin also increases muscle and adipose tissue glucose uptake and decreases hepatic glucose production, and it has antiinflammatory and antiatherogenic effects in rodents.[2,50] Centrally, it activates hypothalamic receptors to stimulate appetite and increase energy expenditure, and may act in a reciprocal manner with leptin to regulate energy stores under different environmental and nutritional conditions.[50]

In humans, plasma adiponectin (particularly HMW forms) paradoxically decreases with obesity, and several studies have shown a negative correlation between body weight and total adiponectin concentration in dogs and cats.[20,56–58] In cats, attempts have also been made to characterize adiponectin multimer concentrations, and 2 recent studies showed preferential decreases in the HMW forms with increasing body mass.[59,60] However, in contrast with several previous results, these studies failed to find a correlation between total adiponectin concentration and body weight. Discrepancies between studies regarding the effect of obesity on adiponectin in dogs and cats[20,36,56–60] may be owing to differences in patient population, timeline and degree of obesity, or assay sensitivity and performance.

CHANGES IN ENERGY REGULATION IN OBESITY

Despite their elevated leptin concentrations, obese cats do not show increases in energy expenditure commensurate with adiposity in progressive obesity. In a longitudinal study of feline weight gain, although energy expenditure (measured as heat production during indirect calorimetry) increased with increasing body mass, the increase tapered off as the cats approached 100% gain over their lean body weight.[23] A previous study had also shown decreased energy expenditure per metabolic body size in obese compared with lean cats,[61] although the appropriate method of normalizing energy expenditure in animals with different body composition remains a matter of debate.[62,63] Additionally, a decreased caloric requirement for weight maintenance has been shown after weight loss programs in cats and dogs, suggesting an increase in metabolic efficiency that must be surmounted during the weight maintenance period.[64,65] Thus far, a mechanism for changes in energy metabolism that occur with obesity in pets has not been determined, but these changes may contribute to difficulties with weight loss in obese pets.

OBESITY AND OTHER ENDOCRINE ABNORMALITIES

In humans, obesity is associated with mildly increased serum thyroid-stimulating hormone and triiodothyronine concentrations,[66] increased serum growth hormone (but not insulinlike growth factor-1) concentrations,[67] increased circulating concentrations of angiotensinogen, renin, angiotensin-converting enzyme, and aldosterone,[68] and low androgen levels.[67] The functional implications of most of these changes are not well-understood, although obesity is known to interfere with reproductive capability,[69] and changes in the components of the renin-angiotensin-aldosterone system are thought to contribute to oxidative stress and altered glucose metabolism.[68]

In dogs and cats, information about the effects of obesity on these variables is limited. No increase in thyroid-stimulating hormone was found with weight gain in cats, although free T4 was increased with obesity, likely because of increased NEFA concentrations.[70] In obese dogs, total T4 and triiodothyronine were both slightly increased, but there was no change in thyroid-stimulating hormone or free T4.[71] Insulinlike growth factor-1 concentrations have also been reported to increase with development of obesity in dogs.[72] Similar to the human situation, the functional significance of such changes is unclear at this time.

OBESITY AND LIPID DISORDERS
Dyslipidemia

As noted, the only consistent abnormality noted on routine biochemical panels in obese, nondiabetic cats compared with lean cats is an increase in serum triglycerides.[34] A study characterizing the serum lipid profiles of obese cats revealed that they have higher proportions of very low-density lipoprotein (VLDL) triglycerides and higher concentrations of small dense low-density lipoproteins than do lean cats.[29] These abnormalities are similar to the dyslipidemia seen in insulin-resistant rodents and in obese humans with the metabolic syndrome[73,74]; in humans, they are associated with increased risk of cardiovascular disease (atherosclerosis) and stroke.

Unlike the human situation, dyslipidemia in obese cats does not seem to confer a risk of atherosclerosis or other cardiovascular consequences, as evidenced by the absence of atherosclerosis in long-term obese cats on postmortem examination (Hoenig and Gal, unpublished data, 2011). This may be owing to the lack of concurrent changes in circulating inflammatory markers and cytokines in obese cats.[23] Adipose tissue in obese humans and rodents is infiltrated by macrophages with a proinflammatory phenotype.[75,76] TNF-α and IL-6 may be released either from these macrophages or from dysfunctional adipocytes, resulting in local and systemic elevations of inflammatory markers[76,77] and promotion of vascular lesions. In cats, obesity-induced macrophage infiltration has not been reported, and obese cats do not have either elevated plasma concentrations of TNF-α, IL-1, or IL-6, or decreased concentrations of circulating antioxidants (associated with oxidative stress).[23] However, obese cats do have increased TNF-α messenger RNA in adipose tissue,[78] suggesting inflammatory mediators may still participate in feline insulin resistance by acting locally.[23]

Elevated plasma triglyceride and cholesterol concentrations, with increased triglyceride and cholesterol in all lipoprotein fractions, have been reported in chronically obese dogs.[79] Some studies have found increases in serum concentrations of inflammatory markers with canine obesity (eg, increased C-reactive protein and IL-6, but not TNF-α or IL-8[80]), and some, but not all, studies have found decreases in such markers and other cytokines (cysteine-rich protein 1, monocyte chemoattractant protein-1, haptoglobin, TNF-α) with weight loss.[15,36,54,81] As is the case for adipocytokines, differences among studies may be related to the assays used or characteristics of the patient population.

Fat Distribution and Tissue Lipid Accumulation

Insulin resistance of obesity has been associated not only with total fat mass, but also with the distribution of triglycerides within the body and within tissues. A loss of insulin sensitivity has been associated particularly with triglyceride deposition in the abdomen (abdominal subcutaneous and intraabdominal), muscle, and liver. There are several methods available to determine fat mass in animals or humans. Most of them give an assessment of whole body fat, but few are sensitive enough to provide the exact localization of fat within the body. Among the latter, however, are MRI and MR spectroscopy (MRS).

- MRI and MRS have their origin in nuclear MR. Both techniques are noninvasive. MRI is used to produce anatomic images, whereas MRS provides chemical and physiologic information. Nuclear MR uses the fact that every molecule is composed of atoms that have nuclei with magnetic properties associated with nuclear "spin." When placed into a strong magnetic field, the spins of these nuclei absorb energy at a specific radio wave frequency and they precess around the larger magnetic field at these specific frequencies. This action is called resonance. The resonance frequency for a given nucleus depends not only on the applied magnetic field, but also on the magnetic field created by the circulating electrons. This allows mapping of molecules because each chemically distinct atom in a molecule will give a different resonance (for review see Webb and Aliev[82]).

- Nuclear MR has been used extensively in rodents and humans. We have used it in cats to investigate changes associated with obesity, in particular location of fat deposits and intracellular triglyceride (as well as metabolic pathways related to EGP as mentioned). It has also been used in dogs for research purposes.

Abdominal fat distribution

There is some controversy as to whether the intraabdominal or subcutaneous abdominal fat is more important in the development of insulin resistance,[83,84] and the quantification of fat at these locations and its correlation with insulin signaling has been an active area of research for many years. It is thought that intraabdominal fat leads to an increased flux of adipocytokines and hormones,[85,86] and has increased lipolytic activity, which negatively influences insulin signaling.[87] Others suggest that abdominal subcutaneous fat is more critical for changes in insulin sensitivity,[88] in part owing to its greater volume.

We investigated abdominal fat distribution in lean cats, and also in obese cats before and after weight loss. With MRI, it was seen that the total fat mass, as expected, was much larger in obese cats than in lean cats. However, in contrast with humans, the abdominal fat mass of cats was equally distributed between abdominal subcutaneous tissue and the intraabdominal area and there was no gender difference. Abdominal subcutaneous, intraabdominal, and total fat correlated significantly with insulin sensitivity. Weight loss was associated with similar fat loss of subcutaneous and intraabdominal fat and led to improved insulin sensitivity, suggesting that fat at both locations influences insulin sensitivity and that fat distribution is not a cause for the greater risk of male cats to develop diabetes.[20]

We are not aware of a similar study in dogs, although 1 investigation using computed tomography showed equal increments of visceral and subcutaneous adipose tissue in dogs during weight gain.[89]

Lipid accumulation in muscle

Using MRS, we investigated the lipid content in muscle in lean and obese cats and found that triglyceride deposits were significantly higher in obese insulin-resistant cats in the intracellular and extramyocellular space. Excess lipid in both sites was highly correlated with decreased insulin sensitivity.[27] This is different from what has been found in adult humans, where the intramyocellular deposit determines the effectiveness of insulin.[90]

In children, similar to cats, fat deposits in both seem to play a role.[91] Our finding that muscle lipoprotein lipase activity and lipoprotein lipase messenger RNA levels were higher in obese cats leading to a significantly higher ratio between muscle and adipose tissue suggests that in the development of obesity a partitioning of fatty acids away from adipose tissue toward muscle tissue is favored.[27] The increased partitioning of fatty acids into muscle tissue is thought to cause insulin resistance because uptake of free fatty acids negatively influences glucose transport.[92] Indeed, as mentioned, decreased GLUT4 expression is an early change in developing obesity in cats, and is evident before overt glucose intolerance is present.[24] However, it is also possible that the increased lipid content in muscle is secondary to the change in glucose uptake. This would allow the use of myocellular lipid as alternative fuel when glucose uptake is low.

Lipid accumulation in the liver

Using MRS and also a chemical assay, we have also found that hepatic triglyceride content was higher in obese than in lean cats (**Fig. 3**).[93] Although a clear cause/effect relation of hepatic lipids and insulin sensitivity has not been identified, it has been suggested that insulin action in the liver is in part determined by the intrahepatic

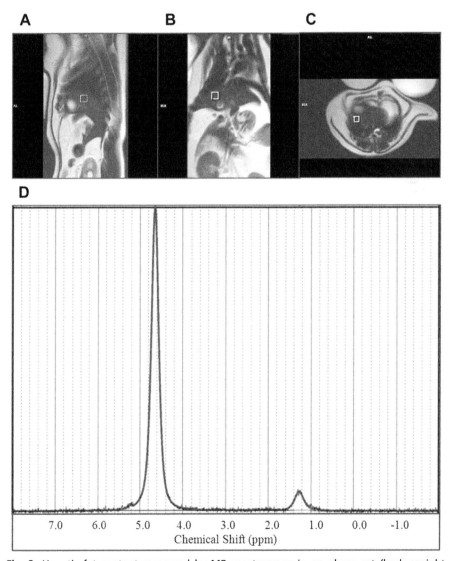

Fig. 3. Hepatic fat content measured by MR spectroscopy in an obese cat (body weight 6.5 kg; liver triglyceride 6.5%). Figure shows a representative spectrum (*D*), with corresponding localizing scans and voxel placement (*A*, sagittal view; *B*, dorsal view; *C*, transverse view). (*From* Clark M, Larsen R. Hoenig M. Investigation of 1H MRS for quantification of hepatic triglyceride in lean and obese cats. Res Vet Sci 2013;95(2):679; with permission.)

triglyceride content and increased fat content in the liver leads to lipid peroxidation, hepatocellular degeneration, and necrosis.[94] Some researchers have argued that there is no obvious threshold that separates normal from abnormal hepatic lipid content.[95] However, the fact that the thiazolidinedione drug class leads to an increase in whole body insulin sensitivity[96–99] and a parallel reduction in liver fat[98] points strongly to a role of liver fat in the regulation of insulin sensitivity.

Predisposition of Obese Cats to Hepatic Lipidosis

HL in cats is characterized by marked hepatocellular triglyceride accumulation after a period of partial to complete anorexia[100] and is more common in obese individuals.[101] Its pathogenesis is thought to involve (1) a negative energy balance, (2) induction of hormonal alterations (eg, hypoinsulinemia, elevated glucagon:insulin ratios) that promote excessive peripheral lipolysis, and (3) delivery of high levels of endogenous lipids to the liver.[100–103] Cats with HL have a 3-fold elevation of serum NEFAs relative to control cats,[102] in contrast with cats with anorexia or obesity alone.[27,29,102]

NEFAs delivered to the liver may be disposed of either through transport into mitochondria for beta-oxidation or through re-esterification and storage in cytosolic droplets.[104] A proportion of stored triglyceride is later secreted as VLDL.[105] Although both beta oxidation and VLDL secretion in cats with HL seem to be increased,[106] clearly neither occurs at a rate sufficient to prevent triglyceride accumulation. Some investigators have suggested that this is because of compartmentalization of triglyceride pools in the hepatocyte: triglyceride in vacuoles is destined for VLDL secretion, and whereas rates of both beta-oxidation and VLDL secretion are finite, the capacity for triglyceride storage is not. Thus, excess NEFA delivery may promote excess triglyceride storage, which persists despite maximal beta-oxidation and VLDL secretion.[106] In obese cats, the presence of preexisting liver lipid deposition, possible increased relative exposure of lean tissues to circulating NEFAs, and altered fat metabolism with failure to appropriately sequester lipid, may all play a role in the tendency toward HL when anorexia or food deprivation occurs. However, further study is needed to define more specifically the factors contributing to this condition.

THE "METABOLIC SYNDROME" IN OBESE PETS
Dogs

A recent study of weight loss in client-owned obese dogs proposed the term "obesity-related metabolic dysfunction" to describe a possible canine analogue of human metabolic syndrome. Criteria for this syndrome were a body condition score of 7 or greater on a 9-point scale, and any two of triglycerides greater than 200 mg/dL, cholesterol greater than 300 mg/dL, systolic blood pressure >160 mm Hg, and fasting blood glucose greater than 100 mg/dL or previously diagnosed type 2 DM. Overall, 7 of 35 dogs fulfilled these criteria before weight loss. All plasma triglyceride and cholesterol concentrations above the normal range normalized with weight loss, but other parameters (systolic blood pressure, blood glucose) did not in the majority of dogs in which they were abnormal. No difference in pre–weight loss body composition analysis, weight loss outcome, systolic blood pressure, plasma triglycerides, cholesterol, glucose, or C-reactive protein could be demonstrated between the dogs that fit the criteria for obesity-related metabolic dysfunction and those that did not, but dogs defined as having obesity-related metabolic dysfunction did have higher baseline insulin and lower adiponectin concentrations. The authors concluded that defining dogs based on metabolic status might have some usefulness, but no correlation with outcomes could be made from these data.[15]

Cats

Clearly, obese cats are subject to certain components of the human metabolic syndrome (eg, insulin resistance, dyslipidemia), and it is also tempting to draw a connection between human nonalcoholic fatty liver disease and hepatic lipid accumulation or HL in obese cats. However, although human nonalcoholic fatty liver disease is similar to feline HL in that it involves high circulating NEFAs, which are the source of excess triglyceride in hepatocytes, it differs from the feline syndrome it typically develops in the context of overnutrition rather than anorexia, with insulin levels often remaining elevated. In addition, it has a significant necroinflammatory component that seems to be absent in obese cats with liver lipid accumulation.[107] The absence of hepatic inflammation in obese cats with elevated liver lipid may be related to the apparent overall lack of a systemic inflammatory response to obesity in this species. Additionally, as discussed elsewhere in this paper, they do not seem to be prone to preferential deposition of visceral over subcutaneous fat, unlike humans with metabolic syndrome and central adiposity, or to obesity-related cardiovascular disease (eg, atherosclerosis). As is the case for dogs, no system of classification has been developed for cats that can predict those most at risk for obesity-related metabolic complications.

SUMMARY

Obesity in pet dogs and cats results in numerous metabolic abnormalities, just as it does in other mammalian species studied. These include insulin resistance, altered adipokine secretion, changes in metabolic rate, abnormal lipid metabolism, and fat accumulation in visceral organs. Because of these changes, obese cats are predisposed to endocrine and metabolic disorders such as DM and HL, and a connection likely also exists between obesity and DM in dogs. Unlike humans with obesity-induced metabolic disease, however, cats do not have consistent evidence of systemic inflammation with obesity, and, perhaps as a result, are not subject to atherosclerosis. No system has yet been developed to identify those obese pets that are at greatest risk for development of obesity-associated metabolic diseases, and further study in this area is needed.

REFERENCES

1. Klausner J. Banfield Pet Hospital State of Pet Health 2011 Report. Available at: www.banfield.co/Banfield/media/PDF/Downloads/soph/Banfield-State-of-Pet-Health-Report-2011.pdf. Accessed January 11, 2016.
2. Kershaw EE, Flier JS. Adipose tissue as an endocrine organ. J Clin Endocrinol Metab 2004;89(6):2548–56.
3. Guyton AC, Hall JE. Insulin, glucagon, and diabetes mellitus. In: Guyton AC, Hall JE, editors. Textbook of medical physiology. 10th edition. Philadelphia: W.B. Saunders Company; 2000. p. 884–98.
4. Yamauchi T, Kamon J, Waki H, et al. The fat-derived hormone adiponectin reverses insulin resistance associated with both lipoatrophy and obesity. Nat Med 2001;7:941–6.
5. Huang-Doran I, Sleigh A, Rochford JJ, et al. Lipodystrophy: metabolic insights from a rare disorder. J Endocrinol 2010;207(3):245–55.

6. Maury E, Brichard SM. Adipokine dysregulation, adipose tissue inflammation and metabolic syndrome. Mol Cell Endocrinol 2010;314:1–16.

7. Lam DW, LeRoith D. Metabolic syndrome [Internet]. In: DeGroot LJ, Beck-Peccoz P, Chrousos G, et al, editors. Endotext. South Dartmouth (MA): MDText.co, Inc; 2000. Accessed January 5, 2016.

8. Hosogai N, Fukuhara A, Oshima K, et al. Adipose tissue hypoxia in obesity and its impact on adipokine dysregulation. Diabetes 2007;56:901–11.

9. Goossens GH. The role of adipose tissue dysfunction in the pathogenesis of obesity-related insulin resistance. Physiol Behav 2008;94:206–18.

10. Yin X, Lanz IR, Swain JM, et al. Adipocyte mitochondrial function is reduced in human obesity independent of fat cell size. J Clin Endocrinol Metab 2014;99(2): E209–16.

11. Samuel VT, Petersen KF, Shulman GI. Insulin resistance. In: Arias IM, Wolkoff A, Boyer J, et al, editors. The liver: biology and pathobiology. 5th edition. Chichester (United Kingdom): John Wiley & Sons Ltd.; 2009. p. 472–83.

12. McQuaid SE, Hodson L, Neville MJ, et al. Downregulation of adipose tissue fatty acid trafficking in obesity: a driver for ectopic fat deposition? Diabetes 2011; 60(1):47–55.

13. Bays H. Central obesity as a clinical marker of adiposopathy; increased visceral adiposity as a surrogate marker for global fat dysfunction. Curr Opin Endocrinol Diabetes Obes 2014;21(5):345–51.

14. Jahanosouz C. Adipocyte dysfunction, inflammation, and insulin resistance in obesity. In: Kurian M, Wolfe BM, Ikramuddin S, editors. Metabolic syndrome and diabetes. New York: Springer Science and Business Media; 2016. p. 61–80. Accessed January 5, 2016.

15. Tvarijonaviciute A, Ceron JJ, Holden SL, et al. Obesity-related metabolic dysfunction in dogs: a comparison with the human metabolic syndrome. BMC Vet Res 2012;8:147.

16. Saltiel AR, Kahn CR. Insulin signalling and the regulation of glucose and lipid metabolism. Nature 2001;414:799–806.

17. Conte C, Fabbrini E, Kars M, et al. Multiorgan insulin sensitivity in lean and obese subjects. Diabetes Care 2012;35:1316–21.

18. Buse JB, Polonsky KS, Burant CF. Type 2 diabetes mellitus. In: Larsen PR, Kronenberg HM, Melmed S, et al, editors. Williams textbook of endocrinology. 10th edition. Pennsylvania: Elsevier Science; 2003. p. 1427–84.

19. Kahn SE, Prigeon RL, McCulloch DK, et al. Quantification of the relationship between insulin sensitivity and beta-cell function in human subjects. Evidence for a hyperbolic function. Diabetes 1993;42:1663–72.

20. Hoenig M, Thomaseth K, Waldron M, et al. Insulin sensitivity, fat distribution and adipocytokine response to different diets in lean, and obese cats before and after weight loss. Am J Physiol 2007;292:R227–34.

21. Biourge V, Nelson RW, Feldman EC, et al. Effect of weight gain and subsequent weight loss on glucose tolerance and insulin response in healthy cats. J Vet Intern Med 1997;11(2):86–91.

22. Hoenig M, Hall G, Ferguson D, et al. A feline model of experimentally induced islet amyloidosis. Am J Pathol 2000;157(6):2143–50.

23. Hoenig M, Pach N, Thomaseth K, et al. Cats differ from other species in their cytokine and antioxidant enzyme response when developing obesity. Obesity (Silver Spring) 2013;21:E407–14.

24. Brennan CL, Hoenig M, Ferguson DC. GLUT4 but not GLUT1 expression decreases early in the development of feline obesity. Domest Anim Endocrinol 2004;26:291–301.
25. Mattheuws D, Rottiers R, Baeyens D, et al. Glucose tolerance and insulin response in obese dogs. J Am Anim Hosp Assoc 1984;20:287–93.
26. Bailhache E, Nguyen P, Krempf M, et al. Lipoproteins abnormalities in obese insulin-resistant dogs. Metabolism 2003;52(5):559–64.
27. Wilkins CE, Long RC Jr, Waldron M, et al. Assessment of the influence of fatty acids on indices of insulin sensitivity and myocellular lipid content by use of magnetic resonance spectroscopy in cats. Am J Vet Res 2004;65:1090–9.
28. Kley S, Caffall Z, Tittle E, et al. Development of a feline proinsulin immunoradiometric assay and a feline proinsulin enzyme-linked immunosorbent assay (ELISA): A novel application to examine beta cell function in cats. Domest Anim Endocrinol 2008;34(3):311–8.
29. Jordan E, Kley S, Le N-A, et al. Dyslipidemia in obese cats. Domest Anim Endocrinol 2008;35(3):290–9.
30. Hoenig M, Jordan ET, Glushka J, et al. Effect of macronutrients, age, and obesity on 6 and 24-hour post-prandial glucose metabolism in cats. Am J Physiol Regul Integr Comp Physiol 2011;301:R1798–807.
31. Weir GC, Laybutt DR, Kaneto H, et al. Beta cell adaptation and decompensation during the progression of diabetes. Diabetes 2001;50(Suppl 1):S154–9.
32. Saisho Y, Butler AE, Manesso E, et al. Beta cell mass and turnover in humans: effects of obesity and aging. Diabetes Care 2013;36(1):111–7.
33. Ader M, Stefanovski D, Kim SP, et al. Hepatic insulin clearance is the primary determinant of insulin sensitivity in the normal dog. Obesity (Silver Spring) 2014;22:1238–45.
34. Hoenig M, Traas A, Schaeffer D. Evaluation of routine blood profiles, fructosamine, thyroxine, insulin, and proinsulin concentrations in client-owned lean, overweight, obese, and diabetic cats. J Am Vet Med Assoc 2013;243(9):1302–9.
35. Hoenig M, Pach N, Thomaseth K, et al. Evaluation of long-term glucose homeostasis in lean and obese cats by use of continuous glucose monitoring. Am J Vet Res 2012;73(7):1100–6.
36. German AJ, Hervera M, Hunter L, et al. Improvement in insulin resistance and reduction in plasma inflammatory adipokines after weight loss in obese dogs. Domest Anim Endocrinol 2009;37:214–26.
37. Panciera DL, Thomas CB, Eicker SW, et al. Epizootiologic patterns of diabetes mellitus in cats: 333 cases (1980-1986). J Am Vet Med Assoc 1990;197(11):1504–8.
38. Scarlett JM, Donoghue S. Associations between body condition and disease in cats. J Am Vet Med Assoc 1998;212(11):1725–31.
39. Prentki M, Nolan CJ. Islet ß-cell failure in type 2 diabetes. J Clin Invest 2006; 116(7):1802–10.
40. Matsuda M, Kawasaki F, Mikami Y, et al. Rescue of beta-cell exhaustion by diazoxide after the development of diabetes mellitus in rats with streptozotocin-induced diabetes. Eur J Pharmacol 2002;453:141–8.
41. Henson MS, Hegstad-Davies RL, Wang Q, et al. Evaluation of plasma islet amyloid polypeptide and serum glucose and insulin concentrations in nondiabetic cats classified by body condition score and in cats with naturally occurring diabetes mellitus. Am J Vet Res 2011;72(8):1052–8.
42. Lorenzo A, Razzaboni B, Weir GC, et al. Pancreatic islet cell toxicity of amylin associated with type-2 diabetes mellitus. Nature 1994;368(6473):756–60.

43. O'Brien TD. Pathogenesis of feline diabetes mellitus. Mol Cell Endocrinol 2002; 197:213–9.
44. O'Brien TD, Hayden DW, Johnson KH, et al. Immunohistochemical morphometry of pancreatic endocrine cells in diabetic, normoglycaemic glucose-intolerant and normal cats. J Comp Pathol 1986;96:357–69.
45. Yano BL, Hayden DW, Johnson KH. Feline insular amyloid: incidence in adult cats with no clinicopathologic evidence of overt diabetes mellitus. Vet Pathol 1981;18:310–5.
46. Henson MS, O'Brien TD. Feline models of type 2 diabetes mellitus. ILAR J 2006; 47(3):234–42.
47. Weyer C, Bogardus C, Mott DM, et al. The natural history of insulin secretory dysfunction and insulin resistance in the pathogenesis of type 2 diabetes mellitus. J Clin Invest 1999;104(6):787–94.
48. Hoenig M, Dawe DL. A qualitative assay for beta cell antibodies. Preliminary results in dogs with diabetes mellitus. Vet Immunol Immunopathol 1992;32: 195–203.
49. Mattheuws D, Rottiers R, Kaneko JJ, et al. Diabetes mellitus in dogs: relationship of obesity to glucose tolerance and insulin response. Am J Vet Res 1984;45(1): 98–103.
50. Galic S, Oakhill J, Steinberg GR. Adipose tissue as an endocrine organ. Mol Cell Endocrinol 2010;316:129–39.
51. Zhang Y, Proenca R, Maffel M, et al. Positional cloning of the mouse obese gene and its human homologue. Nature 1994;372:425–32.
52. Appleton DJ, Rand JS, Sunvold GD. Plasma leptin concentration in cats: reference range, effect of weight gain and relationship with adiposity as measured by dual energy X-ray absorptiometry. J Feline Med Surg 2000;2:191–9.
53. Ishioka K, Hosoya K, Kitagawa H, et al. Plasma leptin concentration in dogs: effects of body condition score, age, gender, and breeds. Res Vet Sci 2007;82: 11–35.
54. Wakshlag JJ, Struble AM, Levine CB, et al. The effects of weight loss on adipokines and markers of inflammation in dogs. Br J Nutr 2011;106:S11–4.
55. Nishii N, Nodake H, Takasu M, et al. Postprandial changes in leptin concentration of cerebrospinal fluid in dogs during development of obesity. Am J Vet Res 2006;67:2006–11.
56. Kley S, Hoenig M, Glushka J, et al. The impact of obesity, sex, and diet on hepatic glucose production in cats. Am J Physiol Regul Integr Comp Physiol 2009;296:R936–43.
57. Park H-J, Lee S-E, Oh J-H, et al. Leptin, adiponectin, and serotonin levels in lean and obese dogs. BMC Vet Res 2014;10:113.
58. Ishioka K, Omachi A, Sagawa M, et al. Canine adiponectin: cDNA structure, mRNA expressin in adipose tissues and reduced plasma levels in obesity. Res Vet Sci 2005;80:127–32.
59. Bjornvad CR, Rand JS, Tan HY, et al. Obesity and sex influence insulin resistance and total and multimer adiponectin levels in adult neutered domestic shorthair client-owned cats. Domest Anim Endocrinol 2014;47:55–64.
60. Witzel AJ, Kirk CA, Kania SA, et al. Relationship of adiponectin and its multimers to metabolic indices in cats during weight change. Domest Anim Endocrinol 2015;53:70–7.
61. Hoenig M, Thomaseth K, Waldron M, et al. Fatty acid turnover, substrate oxidation, and heat production in lean and obese cats during the euglycemic hyper-insulinemic clamp. Domest Anim Endocrinol 2007;32(4):329–38.

62. Arch JRS, Hislop D, Wang SJY, et al. Some mathematical and technical issues in the measurement and interpretation of open-circuit indirect calorimetry in small animals. Int J Obes 2006;30:1322–31.

63. Tschöp MH, Speakman JR, Arch JRS. A guide to analysis of mouse energy metabolism. Nat Methods 2012;9(1):57–63.

64. German AJ, Holden SL, Mather NJ, et al. Low-maintenance energy requirements of obese dogs after weight loss. Br J Nutr 2011;106(Suppl 1):S93–6.

65. Villaverde C, Ramsey JJ, Green AS, et al. Energy restriction results in a mass-adjusted decrease in energy expenditure in cats that is maintained after weight regain. J Nutr 2008;138(5):856–60.

66. Reinehr T. Obesity and thyroid function. Mol Cell Endocrinol 2010;316:165–71.

67. Menucci MB, Burman KD. Endocrine changes in obesity [Internet]. In: DeGroot LJ, Beck-Peccoz P, Chrousos G, et al, editors. Endotext. South Dartmouth (MA): MDText.co, Inc; 2000. Accessed January 5, 2016.

68. Favre GA, Esnault VLM, Van Obberghen E. Modulation of glucose metabolism by the renin-angiotensin-aldosterone system. Am J Physiol Endocrinol Metab 2015;308:E435–49.

69. Rachón D, Teede H. Ovarian function and obesity – interrelationships, impact on women's reproductive lifespan and treatment options. Mol Cell Endocrinol 2010; 316:172–9.

70. Ferguson DC, Caffal Z, Hoenig M. Obesity increases free thyroxine proportionally to nonesterified fatty acid concentrations in adult neutered female cats. J Endocrinol 2007;194(2):267–73.

71. Daminet S, Jeusette I, Duchateau L, et al. Evaluation of thyroid function in obese dogs and in dogs undergoing a weight loss protocol. J Vet Med A Physiol Pathol Clin Med 2003;50:213–8.

72. Gayet C, Bailhache E, Dumon H, et al. Insulin resistance and changes in plasma concentration of TNF alpha, IGF1, and NEFA in dogs during weight gain and obesity. J Anim Physiol Anim Nutr (Berl) 2004;88:157–65.

73. Ginsberg HN, Zhang Y-L, Hernandez-Ono A. Regulation of plasma triglycerides in insulin resistance and diabetes. Arch Med Res 2005;36:232–40.

74. Sørenson LP, Søndergaard E, Nelleman B, et al. Increased VLDL-triglyceride secretion precedes impaired control of endogenous glucose production in obese, normoglycemic men. Diabetes 2011;60:2257–64.

75. Wellen KE, Hotamsligil GS. Inflammation, stress, and diabetes. J Clin Invest 2005;115(5):1111–9.

76. Glass CK, Olefsky JM. Inflammation and lipid signaling in the etiology of insulin resistance. Cell Metab 2012;15:635–45.

77. Park HS, Park JY, Yu R. Relationship of obesity and visceral adiposity with serum concentrations of CRP, TNF-α and IL-6. Diabetes Res Clin Pract 2005;69:29–35.

78. Hoenig M, McGoldrick JB, DeBeer M, et al. Activity and tissue-specific expression of lipases and tumor-necrosis factor -α in lean and obese cats. Domest Anim Endocrinol 2006;30:333–44.

79. Jeusette IC, Lhoest ET, Istasse LP, et al. Influence of obesity on plasma lipid and lipoprotein concentrations in dogs. Am J Vet Res 2005;66(1):81–6.

80. Frank L, Mann S, Levine CB, et al. Increasing body condition score is positively associated with interleukin-6 and monocyte chemoattractant protein-1 in Labrador retrievers. Vet Immunol Immunopathol 2015;167:104–9.

81. Bastien BC, Patil A, Satyaraj E. The impact of weight loss on circulating cytokine in Beagle dogs. Vet Immunol Immunopathol 2015;163:174–82.

82. Webb GA, Schilf W. Nuclear magnetic resonance. In: Webb GA, Aliev AE, editors. Royal society of chemistry; 2003.
83. Abate N, Garg A, Peshock RM, et al. Relationships of generalized and regional adiposity to insulin sensitivity in men. J Clin Invest 1995;96:88–98.
84. Frayn KN. Visceral fat and insulin resistance–causative or correlative? Br J Nutr 2000;83(Suppl 1):S71–7.
85. Coelho M, Oliveira T, Fernandes R. Biochemistry of adipose tissue: an endocrine organ. Arch Med Sci 2013;9:191–200.
86. Silveira LS, Monteiro PA, Antunes Bde M, et al. Intra-abdominal fat is related to metabolic syndrome and non-alcoholic fat liver disease in obese youth. BMC Pediatr 2013;13:115–21.
87. Kim SP, Ellmerer M, Van Citters GW, et al. Primacy of hepatic insulin resistance in the development of the metabolic syndrome induced by an isocaloric moderate-fat diet in the dog. Diabetes 2003;52:2453–60.
88. Baldisserotto M, Damiani D, Cominato L, et al. Subcutaneous fat: a better marker than visceral fat for insulin resistance in obese adolescents. ESPEN J 2013;8(6):e251–5.
89. Adolphe JL, Silver TI, Childs H, et al. Short-term obesity results in detrimental metabolic and cardiovascular changes that may not be reversed with weight loss in an obese dog model. Br J Nutr 2014;112:647–56.
90. Virkamäki A, Korsheninnikova E, Seppälä-Lindroos A, et al. Intramyocellular lipid is associated with resistance to in vivo insulin actions on glucose uptake, antilipolysis, and early insulin signaling pathways in human skeletal muscle. Diabetes 2001;50:2337–43.
91. Sinha R, Dufour S, Peterson KF, et al. Assessment of skeletal muscle triglyceride content by 1H nuclear magnetic resonance spectroscopy in lean and obese adolescents. Diabetes 2002;51:1022–7.
92. Thompson AL, Lim-Fraser MYC, Kraegen EW, et al. Effects of individual fatty acids on glucose uptake and glycogen synthesis in soleus muscle in vitro. Am J Physiol Endocrinol Metab 2000;279(3):E577–84.
93. Clark M, Larsen R, Hoenig M. Investigation of 1H MRS for quantification of hepatic triglyceride in lean and obese cats. Res Vet Sci 2013;95(2):678–80.
94. Hijona E, Hijona L, Arenas JI, et al. Inflammatory mediators of hepatic steatosis. Mediators Inflamm 2010;2010:837419.
95. Fabbrini E, Sullivan S, Klein S. Obesity and nonalcoholic fatty liver disease: Biochemical, metabolic, and clinical implications. Hepatology 2010;51:679–89.
96. Hoenig M, Ferguson DC. Effect of darglitazone on glucose clearance and lipid metabolism in obese cats. Am J Vet Res 2003;64:1409–13.
97. Ikeda H, Taketomi S, Sugiyama Y, et al. Effects of pioglitazone on glucose and lipid metabolism in normal and insulin resistant animals. Arzneimittelforschung 1990;40:156–62.
98. Yki-Jarvinen H. Thiazolidinediones. N Engl J Med 2004;351:1106–18.
99. Clark M, Thomaseth K, Dirikolu L, et al. Effects of pioglitazone on insulin sensitivity and serum lipids in obese cats. J Vet Intern Med 2014;28:166–74.
100. Armstrong PJ, Blanchard G. Hepatic lipidosis in cats. Vet Clin North Am Small Anim Pract 2009;39:599–616.
101. Center SA, Crawford MA, Guida L, et al. A retrospective study of 77 cats with severe hepatic lipidosis: 1975-1990. J Vet Intern Med 1993;7:349–59.
102. Brown B, Mauldin GE, Armstrong J, et al. Metabolic and hormonal alterations in cats with hepatic lipidosis. J Vet Intern Med 2000;14:20–6.

103. Hall JA, Barstad LA, Connor WE. Lipid composition of hepatic and adipose tissues from normal cats and from cats with idiopathic hepatic lipidosis. J Vet Intern Med 1997;11(4):238–42.
104. McGarry JD, Foster DW. Regulation of hepatic fatty acid oxidation and ketone body production. Annu Rev Biochem 1980;49:395–420.
105. Gibbons GF, Wiggins D, Brown AM, et al. Synthesis and function of hepatic very-low-density-lipoprotein. Biochem Soc Trans 2004;32:59–64.
106. Pazak H, Bartges JW, Cornelius LC, et al. Characterization of serum lipoprotein profiles of healthy, adult cats and feline hepatic lipidosis patients. J Nutr 1998; 128:2747S–50S.
107. Ahmed MH, Byrne CD. Current treatment of non-alcoholic fatty liver disease. Diabetes Obes Metab 2009;11:188–95.

Impact of Obesity on Cardiopulmonary Disease

Marjorie L. Chandler, DVM, MS, MANZCVS, MRCVS

KEYWORDS

- Cardiopulmonary • Obesity • Obesity paradox • Cat • Dog • Heart • Respiratory

KEY POINTS

- Obesity has detrimental effects on the heart and lung, including physical effects of fat, increased inflammatory mediators, and neurohormonal effects.
- Epidemiologic studies have not proved that obesity is risk factor for cardiopulmonary disorders in dogs and cats, although many dogs with bronchitis are overweight.
- Weight loss in overweight individuals improves cardiac and respiratory parameters and exercise tolerance.
- Overweight dogs that have already been diagnosed with heart disease live longer than those that are thin or normal weight, but this is possibly due to other factors rather than a benefit of body fat.
- Obesity in dogs with obstructive airway disorders is recognized to increase disease severity and these dogs should be put on a weight loss program.

INTRODUCTION

Heart failure is the pathophysiologic state occurring when the heart's ability to eject or receive blood is impaired, resulting in clinical signs that may include increased respiratory effort, coughing, wheezing, ascites, exercise intolerance, cyanosis, and syncope. Heart failure can result from impairment of the myocardium, heart valves, or pericardium or is due to increased peripheral resistance, such as occurs with hypertension. The heart responds to increased workload and increased wall stress by remodeling, and remodeling results in cardiac hypertrophy. This initially normalizes wall stress but eventually an exhaustion phase occurs. This phase is characterized by death of cardiomyocytes, development of myocardial fibrosis, ventricular dilation, and reduced cardiac output. Pathologic remodeling, as opposed to physiologic remodeling, which occurs due to exercise, is often irreversible and reduces systolic or diastolic function.[1]

Neurohormonal changes in heart failure include an increased activity of adrenergic nervous system, activation of the renin-angiotensin-aldosterone system, and

The author has nothing to disclose.
Vets Now Referrals, 123-145 North Street, Glasgow G3 7DA, Scotland
E-mail address: chandlermarge05@gmail.com

Vet Clin Small Anim 46 (2016) 817–830
http://dx.doi.org/10.1016/j.cvsm.2016.04.005
0195-5616/16/$ – see front matter © 2016 Elsevier Inc. All rights reserved.

increased expression of proinflammatory cytokines, including tumor necrosis factor α (TNF-α), interleukin (IL)-1, and IL-6. Heart failure progression is affected by excessive responses of these systems, and dogs and cats have shown similar neuroendocrine changes.[1]

DOES OBESITY HAVE AN EFFECT ON HEART DISEASE?
Human

In humans, large studies have demonstrated that increased body mass index (BMI) is an independent risk factor for heart failure.[2–4] The BMI is body weight in kilograms divided by height in square meters and provides an estimate of human body condition. Overweight and obesity are associated with increased rates of hypertension, coronary heart disease, left ventricular hypertrophy, and diabetes, all of which are also important causes of heart failure. Morbid obesity is recognized as causing a form of cardiomyopathy characterized by chronic volume overload, left ventricular hypertrophy, and left ventricular dilation.[5] Obesity-related hypoventilation and sleep apnea also contribute to heart failure; however, even lesser degrees of overweight result in an increased risk of heart failure independent of these factors. Obese individuals with or without diabetes, especially those with abdominal obesity, may still show metabolic changes or clinical signs consistent with the metabolic syndrome. The metabolic syndrome includes a constellation of clinical changes, which include hypertension, insulin resistance, and atherogenic dyslipidemia with high levels of low-density lipoprotein (LDL) cholesterol and very low-density lipoprotein (VLDL) cholesterol and increased C-reactive protein (CRP). A chronic inflammatory state with elevated cytokines, elevated proinflammatory leptin, and decreased adiponectin is usually present. In humans, the presence of these factors are a risk factor for coronary heart disease, diabetes mellitus, and stroke.[3] (For more information on metabolic syndrome, see Melissa Clark and Margarethe Hoenig's article, "Metabolic Effects of Obesity and Its Interaction with Endocrine Diseases," in this issue.)

Obesity and Heart Disease in Dogs and Cats

The most common cause of heart failure in dogs is valvular disease, especially in small breeds, and it accounts for 75% to 80% of canine cardiac disease.[6] Myocardial disease, especially dilated cardiomyopathy, is also common in dogs.[7] Cardiomyopathies, especially hypertrophic cardiomyopathy (HCM), are the most common causes of heart disease in cats, accounting for more than 60% of feline heart disease.[8]

Obesity does not increase the risk for atherogenic coronary heart disease in dogs and cats as it does in humans. Atherosclerosis is rare in dogs and extremely rare in cats, likely in part due to their relatively high high-density lipoprotein (HDL) to low LDL ratio.[9] Obese cats do have an increase in VLDLs similar to humans but do not develop subsequent hypertension and atherosclerosis, so other antiatherogenic mechanisms may be present.[10,11] Obese dogs show hypertriglyceridemia and hypercholesterolemia, but most of the cholesterol is HDL cholesterol, which is protective against atherosclerosis. The ratio of HDL to LDL cholesterol does not change with weight gain in dogs as it does in humans.[12]

Obesity at the time of diagnosis has not been reported as a risk factor in epidemiologic studies of heart disease in cats and dogs. In 1 study, the median body condition score (BCS) of the dogs with chronic valvular disease was 6 (range of 4–9) whereas the control dogs had a median BCS of 5 (range of 5–7). This difference was not significant ($P = .37$).[13] In another study comparing dogs with heart disease and healthy dogs, there was again no difference in BCS. This study did find an increase in the amount of visceral abdominal obesity in the dogs with heart failure compared with healthy dogs.[14] In more than 50% of dogs with dilated cardiomyopathy, cardiac cachexia (a loss of lean body mass) was reported.[15]

Body weight was not a risk factor in a study of feline HCM,[16] and BCS was also not different for cats with HCM compared with control cats, although the cats with HCM were skeletally larger.[17]

Because obesity is common in adult dogs and cats, it is possible that an overweight or obese body condition had been present previously in pets with heart failure, because weight loss is a common presenting sign; however, this still does not qualify obesity as being a risk factor.

The Effect of Obesity on Heart Function

Obesity is known to have deleterious effects on heart function. Obese dogs have an increase in heart rate and a small to moderate increase in blood pressure compared with lean dogs.[18–21] The increased heart rate may be due to reduced parasympathetic control of heart rate,[18] and the increased blood pressure due to an altered sympathetic control of peripheral vascular resistance.[19] Compared with lean dogs, obese dogs also have increased left ventricular free wall thickness at end diastole and end systole[21] (**Box 1**).

Renin-Angiotensin-Aldosterone System

As well as its role in blood pressure control, the renin-angiotensin system (RAS) plays a role in adipocyte differentiation and metabolism. All components of the RAS are found within fat, and white adipose tissue is a major source of angiotensinogen, second only to the liver.[22] Obesity in humans, rodents, and dogs is associated with activation of the RAS as evidenced by increased levels of circulating angiotensinogen, plasma renin activity, angiotensin-converting enzyme activity, angiotensin II, and aldosterone.[23–25] Increased abdominal visceral fat is associated with a more pronounced activation of the RAS compared with peripheral subcutaneous fat.[22] Overweight dogs have a higher systolic blood pressure than normal weight dogs,[12,26,27] although the difference is not always significant.[26] Obesity has not been reported as a risk factor for hypertension in cats.

With increased fat mass, adipose-derived angiotensinogen increases plasma angiotensinogen concentrations, resulting in more angiotensin II. Increases in

---

Box 1
Potential effects of obesity on the cardiovascular system

Increased heart rate

Hypertension—effect possibly small in dogs

Increased left ventricular free wall thickness at end diastole and end systole

Increased angiotensinogen

Increased levels of RAA activity

Increased sodium retention (due to aldosterone)

Increased inflammation, fibrosis, and oxidative stress (due to aldosterone)

Increased pathologic cardiac remodeling

Abbreviation: RAA, renin, angiotensin, and aldosterone.

angiotensin II promote cardiovascular dysfunction by direct vasoconstrictor activity and by increasing renal sodium retention via increased aldosterone release, which can increase blood pressure.[23–25] Aldosterone and renin have been reported as elevated in dogs with obesity-induced hypertension that had been fat on a high-fat diet for 5 weeks.[28] Using eplererone to antagonize the aldosterone decreased hypertension in these dogs. It is also possible that the high-fat diet contributed to hypertension because high-fat diets can cause sodium retention in some species.[29] Weight loss in humans decreases circulating components of the RAS,[30] and weight loss has been shown to decrease blood pressure in obese dogs.[31]

As well as its effects on the vasculature, aldosterone is a mediator of inflammation, fibrosis, and oxidative stress and is involved in the pathologic cardiac remodeling. Serum aldosterone and plasma renin are often elevated in dogs with congestive heart failure due to mitral regurgitation or dilated cardiomyopathy and in cats with restrictive or HCM.[1] The production of RAS components by adipocytes is exacerbated during obesity.[32] In obese rats, the imbalance of the RAS system is thought to be due to oxidative stress.[33] Like rats, obese dogs have increases in oxidative stress,[34] although the situation is less clear in cats.[35]

Adiponectin

The effects of the adipokine (adiponectin) include improved insulin sensitivity and anti-inflammatory properties. It is generally decreased with obesity and increased in lean individuals. There has been some controversy about the decreasing of adiponectin in obese dogs. Some studies have shown a decrease in adiponectin in obese dogs[36–38] and 1 did not show this decrease.[39] It was speculated that obesity might decrease adiponectin in intact but not in neutered dogs.[39]

Adiponectin has been shown to be decreased in obese cats.[40] Decreases in adiponectin in humans is more severe with increased visceral abdominal fat than with increased subcutaneous fat,[22] and the adiponectin gene expression in cats is also greater in visceral compared with subcutaneous fat.[40]

The decrease in adiponectin with increased fat, especially visceral fat, may be due to increased proinflammatory cytokines and increased reactive oxygen species, although in 1 study on canine adipocytes there was little effect on adiponectin production with the application of the inflammatory mediators TNF-α and lipopolysaccharide.[41]

Adiponectin affects cardiovascular function and may have a palliative effect on pathologic cardiac remodeling after myocardial infarction.[42] The cardiovascular effects may result from the vasodilator functions of adiponectin.[43] Adiponectin increases expression of endothelial nitric oxide synthase and prostacyclin synthase, both of which promote vasorelaxation[44] and decrease the cardiac afterload.[45] Adiponectin also has anti-inflammatory and antiatherogenic properties, which may occur via its ability to suppress TNF-α production by macrophages, suppress myelomonocytic progenitor cell growth, and induce apoptosis.[46] (For further discussion of regulation of adiponectin and its systemic effects, see Beth Hamper's article, "Current Topics in Canine and Feline Obesity" and Melissa Clark and Margarethe Hoenig's article, "Metabolic Effects of Obesity and Its Interaction with Endocrine Diseases," in this issue.)

Metabolic and Biomarker Changes in Weight Loss

In obese humans, markers of inflammation and pro-inflammatory adipokines have been shown to decrease with weight loss. These changes are associated with a decreased risk of cardiovascular disease.[47–49]

A study has shown decreases in the acute-phase proteins haptoglobin and CRP and improving trends in TNF-α after weight loss in overweight dogs.[49] Another study of weight loss in female beagles showed a decrease in serum total cholesterol (both HDL and LDL) and triglycerides but no change in acute-phase proteins.[50] In this study, adiponectin did increase after weight loss. In 25 client-owned overweight dogs on a weight loss program, the acute-phase reactant CRP decreased significantly after weight loss; however, there was no significant increase in adiponectin.[51] Another study showed that although adiponectin was higher in lean dogs and decreased with weight gain, after subsequent weight loss to the original body weights, the adiponectin remained low.[26]

Obesity Effect on Heart Size and Rate

Eighteen neutered female dogs that gained weight on a high-fat diet for 12 weeks developed concentric cardiac hypertrophy, although in the trial period there was no evidence of systolic or diastolic dysfunction, possibly due to the short duration of the obesity.[52] The cardiac hypertrophy in these dogs was reversed within 13 weeks of weight loss. The dogs, which were exercised, had less decrease in cardiac hypertrophy compared with those without exercise; however, exercise is known to stimulate physiologic ventricular hypertrophy. A study of 8 neutered beagles also showed an increased left ventricular wall thickness after weight gain, which was especially associated with visceral fat.[26]

Weight Loss Effects on the Heart

Heart rate also increases with weight gain and normalizes after weight loss.[20,52,53] The increase in left ventricular wall thickness due to obesity also decreases with weight loss in dogs.[26]

Owners often report a subjective improvement in activity after overweight dogs lose weight. In 15 previously overweight dogs, there was an increase in voluntary physical activity of 1.5 hours per day after weight loss.[20] Another study of overweight beagles showed a significant improvement in distance walked during the 6 minute walk test.[54] These dogs also had a subjective improvement in demeanor after weight loss.

The Obesity Paradox and Survival Times

Because of the increased risk of heart disease in humans, it seems that obesity would be associated with a worse survival rate for canine and feline heart failure patients; however, studies have shown that obesity may be associated with better outcomes after a diagnosis of heart failure, a phenomenon, termed the *obesity paradox* or *reverse epidemiology*.[2] Several large human studies have looked at the impact of BMI on mortality in heart patients; most have shown a significant improvement in survival with increased BMI, although in 1 study the benefit was noted at 1 and 2 years but not at a 5-year follow-up.[55] Some studies have shown that in more marked obesity (BMI >35 kg/m^2) there was no improvement in survival.[56] Nearly all studies show an improvement in overweight compared with cachexic patients.

In dogs and cats, obesity does not increase the risk of coronary heart disease, but, as discussed previously, it can have an adverse effect on cardiopulmonary function and blood pressure,[57] so weight loss may be recommended for obese dogs with increased risk of heart failure, such as high-risk breeds. One study in dogs with heart failure that gained, lost, or maintained body weight showed a difference in survival among dogs, with the dogs that gained weight surviving the longest.[57] Oddly, in this study, dogs that lost weight also lived longer than those who maintained their weight. The emaciated dogs with a BCS of 1 to 2 of 9 had the shortest survival time, with the obese dogs (BCS 8–9/9) living the longest; however, there were few dogs in these bottom and top categories and the comparison between BCS and survival was not statistically significant. The overweight dogs (BCS 6–7/9) did outlive the ideal (5/9) BCS dogs.

A study of 101 cats with heart failure due to cardiomyopathy showed that cats with the highest and lowest body weights had reduced survival times compared with those with intermediate body weight. There was no statistically significant association between BCS and survival even though the pattern was similar to that for body weight.[58]

In some human studies, moderate overweight body condition seemed to confer a survival benefit for heart disease, but patients with morbid obesity (BMI >35 mg/kg^2) had worse outcomes than those of normal weight or mild obesity.[59] A U-shaped curve by BMI may exist, similar to that in the feline study, where mortality is greatest in cachectic patients, lower in normal weight or mildly obese, and higher again in severely obese.[59]

Obese human heart patients may be diagnosed earlier due to dyspnea, edema, or other respiratory signs or poor exercise tolerance, which may not be due to severe heart failure. This could mean that these obese patients have healthier hearts than nonobese patients at the time of diagnosis, leading to an apparent longer survival.[56]

Lower BMI and a lower BCS in dogs and cats may reflect the presence of comorbid diseases, which could shorten survival time.[59] These comorbidities contribute to a state of malnutrition and shorter survival. Those patients who maintain or gain weight after diagnosis of their disease may be those who have a better response to treatment or fewer comorbid diseases. The neurohormonal alterations in obesity, for example, plasma adrenaline and renin concentrations, may favor a longer survival in some individuals.[55]

DOES OBESITY AFFECT PULMONARY FUNCTION AND RESPIRATORY DISEASES?
Effects of Obesity on Airway Function and Bronchial Disease

Humans
In humans, obesity causes an increased work of breathing, respiratory muscle inefficiency, decreased respiratory compliance, and increased demand for ventilation. There is a decreased functional residual capacity and expiratory reserve volume, decreased ventilation to perfusion ratio (V/Q) mismatch, and chronic hypoxia.[60] Obesity is known to lead to obstructive sleep apnea syndrome (OSAS), obesity hypoventilation syndrome, and increased airway sensitivity. The increased airway sensitivity may be related to the development of asthma.[61] There is also increased risk of pneumonia, venous thrombosis, embolism, and possibly pulmonary hypertension. Human patients with chronic bronchitis are likely to be obese (**Box 2**). Obesity may play a significant role in the pathogenesis of pulmonary diseases through the increased proinflammatory mediators.

Dogs
Like humans, dogs with chronic bronchitis are often overweight although the cause and effect are not well described.[62] In 36 dogs, obesity did not seem to influence airway function, diffusion capacity of carbon monoxide, or arterial blood gas variables. With hyperpnea, the expiratory specific airway resistance was greater in obese than in nonobese dogs, and the functional residual capacity was lower, although the difference was not significant.[63]

In lean versus obese geriatric dogs without evidence of cardiac or respiratory disease, obese dogs had a significantly lower median partial pressure of oxygen in arterial blood (Pao_2) (80.8 mm Hg; range, 62.8–95.6) than normal dogs (85.4 mm Hg;

Box 2
Potential respiratory system consequences of obesity
Decreased compliance due to chest wall restriction from fat
Increased airway resistance
Increased work of breathing
Respiratory muscle dysfunction
V/Q mismatch
Decreased expiratory reserve volume
Increased respiratory rate
Reduced tidal volume
Decreased Pao_2, especially with exercise
Increased risk of obstructive sleep apnea
Obesity hypoventilation syndrome
Increased risk of bronchitis
Increased risk of pneumonia (human)
Possible relationship to asthma (human)

range, 77.8–94.2). The difference between the alveolar and arterial oxygen ($P[A-a]o_2$) was significantly higher for obese dogs. Obese dogs had significantly greater intrathoracic fat deposition (IFD) than lean dogs. Dogs with moderate IFD had significantly lower Pao_2, and those with mild and moderate IFD had significantly higher $P(A-a)o_2$ than lean dogs. This study concluded that obesity, resulting in IFD, together with ageing, is associated with decreased Pao_2 and increased $P(A-a)o_2$.[64] In 6 beagles that were induced to become obese, the tidal volume per kg body weight was decreased and respiratory rate increased significantly.[65]

In 12 overweight dogs that lost weight, there was no difference in resting arterial blood gas results before and after weight loss, although compared with overweight and normal weight dogs, obese dogs had a lower blood oxygen saturation based on pulse oximetry, especially at the end of a 6-minute walk.[54]

Another study of 8 obese dogs with chronic respiratory disease also reported hypoxemia to be common. After an average weight loss of 12%, there was an improvement in arterial blood gas parameters and in clinical signs of coughing panting, respiratory noise, and exercise tolerance.[66]

Cats

Feline bronchial disease is a common inflammatory disease of the lower airways. A study of 13 obese and 32 normal-weight client-owned cats with natural bronchial disease were evaluated for respiratory function using barometric whole-body plethysmography, a noninvasive pulmonary function test. This test showed no differences in pulmonary function parameters based on body condition.[67]

Another study of overweight versus normal weight cats also showed no significant differences in respiratory parameters, including tidal volume, expiratory and inspiratory times and peak pressures, respiratory rate, partial pressure of end-tidal CO_2 and Pao_2. There was a nonsignificantly higher mean Pao_2 (88.1 mm Hg) in the normal weight cats compared with the overweight cats (72 mm Hg).[68] Conversely, a different study of obese versus nonobese cats did show a significant decrease in tidal volume and minute volume per kilogram body weight and decreased peak inspiratory and expiratory flows per kilogram body weight in obese cats.[69]

Asthma

Humans and rodents

Obesity is a risk factor for asthma in humans and in rodent models. Obese mice have increased airway hyper-responsiveness, a characteristic feature of asthma. Obese mice also respond more to common asthma triggers. The compromised lung mechanics and increased cytokines, acute-phase proteins, and increased oxidative stress present in obesity likely contribute to the relationship between asthma and obesity.[70]

Cats and dogs

No studies have shown a relationship between feline asthma and obesity and 1 study failed to show a significant increase in bronchoconstriction indexes in obese versus nonobese cats.[69] Although dogs can develop eosinophilic bronchopneumopathy (EBP), which in humans is similar to other allergic diseases, such as asthma, canine EBP is not asthma. Although bronchospasm may be present, airway hyper-reactivity is not usually seen in EBP. No relationship to obesity has been reported for canine EBP.[71] Canine airway smooth muscle is less reactive compared with other domestic species, including humans, although reactivity has been reported to increase with obesity.[65]

Respiratory Infections

In obese humans, greater severity of illness due to H1N1 influenza, decreased responsiveness to influenza vaccination, and an increased risk of developing pneumonia after surgery have been reported.[72] Rodents also show impaired immunity to influenza.[72] Conversely, obesity may be protective from death due to pneumonia, potentially another version of the obesity paradox where low BMI results in a higher mortality rate.[73]

Adipokines have a role in innate and adaptive immunity. Adiponectin, which is usually decreased in obesity, plays a role in the uptake of apoptotic cells by macrophages, a critical response for reducing inflammation in the lungs.[72] The decrease in adiponectin could, therefore, contribute to increased pulmonary inflammation.

There has also been discussion of the obesity-promoting effects of some infectious diseases. Canine distemper virus has been reported to cause obesity in mice.[73,74] This is thought to be due to viral infection of the brain, especially the hypothalamus, possibly resulting in leptin resistance and overeating.[74] No studies have examined the effect of obesity on respiratory infections in dogs and cats or the effects of infectious causes of obesity.

Recurrent Airway Obstruction and Obesity

Obstructive airway disorders are highly associated with human obesity. In some brachycephalic breeds which are at high risk for airway obstruction obesity likely also contributes to the disorder (**Fig. 1**). In a study of Norwich terriers with upper airway obstruction, half of them were overweight or obese.[75]

There are several mechanisms by which obesity impairs respiratory function, resulting in exercise intolerance (**Fig. 2**).[76] Obese dogs with obstructive airway disease are at risk during anesthesia and weight loss before elective surgical procedures should be considered.

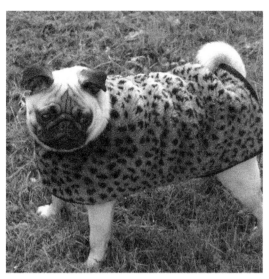

Fig. 1. Brachycephalic breeds are at increased risk for obstructive airway disease, which can be worsened with obesity. (*Courtesy of* Amy Farcas, DVM, MS, DACVN, San Carlos, CA.)

Adipokines may also contribute to the pathophysiology of obstructive airway disease. Leptin levels are frequently increased in obstructive airway disease and in obesity. Leptin resistance, which also occurs in some obese individuals, is thought to contribute to the disease state. Leptin also plays a role in ventilation control and may contribute to hypoventilation in obstructive sleep apnea. The use of continuous positive airway pressure (CPAP) usage reduces leptin levels in dogs with OSAS independent of weight loss, suggesting that leptin is associated with OSAS.[77]

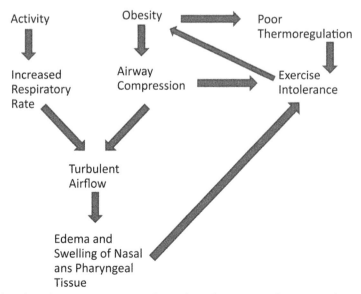

Fig. 2. Flowchart demonstrating interrelationship of respiratory function and obesity.

Adiponectin levels are decreased in OSAS independent of obesity. The magnitude of the decrease correlates with syndrome severity. Because CPAP usage is not associated with subsequent increases in adiponectin, it may be that adiponectin's association with OSAS is related to the obesity.[77]

SUMMARY OF THE RELATIONSHIP OF OBESITY AND CARDIORESPIRATORY DISEASE IN DOGS AND CATS

Although there are detrimental effects of obesity on the heart and lungs, there are few data from epidemiologic studies on obesity as a risk of developing cardiac and pulmonary disorders in dogs and cats. It is probable that increased abdominal fat is especially detrimental as it is in humans, and there is evidence of the negative effects of increased intrathoracic fat. As well as the physical effects of the fat mass, increased inflammatory mediators and neurohormonal effects of obesity likely contribute to cardiopulmonary disorders. The obesity paradox may reflect increased lean tissue and less risk of malnutrition in overweight patients rather than true benefits of extra fat. Weight loss improves cardiac parameters and exercise tolerance in dogs. The obstructive airway disorders are where obesity is best recognized to increase the disease severity.

REFERENCES

1. Sisson DD. Pathophysiology of heart failure. In: Ettinger SJ, Feldman EC, editors. Textbook of veterinary internal medicine. 7th edition. St Louis (MO): Saunders Elsevier; 2010. p. 1143–58.
2. Habbu A, Lakkis NM, Dokainish H. The obesity paradox: fact or fiction. Am J Cardiol 2006;98:944–8.
3. Pi-Sunyer X. The medical risks of obesity. Postgrad Med 2009;121(6):21–33.
4. Kenchaiah S, Evans JC, Levy D, et al. Obesity and the risk of heart disease. N Engl J Med 2002;347(5):305–13.
5. Alpert MA. Obesity cardiomyopathy: pathophysiology and evolution of the clinical syndrome. Am J Med Sci 2001;321:225–36.
6. Olson LH, Haggstrom J, Henrik DP. Acquired valvular heart disease. In: Ettinger SJ, Feldman EC, editors. Textbook of veterinary internal medicine. 7th edition. St Louis (MO): Saunders Elsevier; 2010. p. 1299–319.
7. Meurs KM. Myocardial disease; canine. In: Ettinger SJ, Feldman EC, editors. Textbook of veterinary internal medicine. 7th edition. St Louis (MO): Saunders Elsevier; 2010. p. 1320–7.
8. Macdonald K. Myocardial disease: feline. In: Ettinger SJ, Feldman EC, editors. Textbook of veterinary internal medicine. 7th edition. St Louis (MO): Saunders Elsevier; 2010. p. 1328–41.
9. Boynosky NA, Stokkin L. Atherosclerosis associated with vasculopathic lesions in a golden retriever with hypercholesterolemia. Can Vet J 2014;55(5):484–8.
10. Jordan E, Kley S, Le NA, et al. Dyslipidemia in obese cats. Domest Anim Endocrinol 2008;35(3):290–9.
11. Hoenig M. The cat as a model for human obesity and diabetes. J Diabetes Sci Technol 2012;6(3):525–33.
12. Verkest KR. Is the metabolic syndrome a useful concept in dogs? A review of the evidence. Vet J 2014;199(1):24–30.
13. Freeman LM, Rush JE, Markwell PJ. Effects of dietary modification in dogs with early chronic valvular disease. J Vet Intern Med 2006;20:1116–26.

14. Thengchaisri N, Wutthiwong T, Kaewmokul S, et al. Abdominal obesity is associated with heart disease in dogs. BMC Vet Res 2014;10(1):131.

15. Freeman LM, Rush JE, Kehayias JJ, et al. Nutrition alterations and the effect of fish oil supplementation. J Vet Intern Med 1998;12:440–8.

16. Atkins CE, Gallo MA, Kurzmann ID, et al. Risk factors, clinical signs, and survival in cats with a clinical diagnosis of hypertrophic cardiomyopathy: 74 cases (1985-1989). J Am Vet Med Assoc 1992;201(4):613–8.

17. Yang VK, Freeman LM, Rush JE. Comparisons of morphometric measurements and serum insulin-like growth factor concentration in healthy cats and cats with hypertrophic cardiomyopathy. Am J Vet Res 2008;69(8):1061–6.

18. Van Vliet BN, Hall JE, Mizelle HL, et al. Reduced parasympathetic control of heart rate in obese dogs. Am J Physiol 1995;269(2 Pt 2):H629–37.

19. Truett AA, Borne AT, Poincot MA, et al. Autonomic control of blood pressure and heart rate in obese hypertensive dogs. Am J Physiol 1996;270(3):R541–9.

20. Boutheguard JC, Kelly M, Clety N, et al. Effects of weight loss on heart rate normalization and increase in spontaneous activity in moderately exercised overweight dogs. Int J Appl Res Vet Med 2009;7(4):153–64.

21. Mehlman E, Bright JM, Jeckel K, et al. Echocardiographic evidence of left ventricular hypertrophy in obese dogs. J Vet Intern Med 2013;27(1):62–8.

22. Radin MJ, Sharkey LC, Hylucross BJ. Adipokines: a review of biological and analytical principles and an update in dogs, cats and horses. Vet Clin Pathol 2009;38/2:126–56.

23. Engeli S, Schling P, Gorzelniak K, et al. The adipose-tissue renin-angiotensin-aldosterone system: role in the metabolic syndrome? Int J Biochem Cell Biol 2003;35:807–25.

24. Barton M, Carmona R, Ortmann J, et al. Obesity-associated activation of angiotensin and endothelin in the cardiovascular system. Int J Biochem Cell Biol 2003; 35:826–37.

25. Henegar JR, Bigler SA, Henegar LK, et al. Functional and structural changes in the kidney in the early stages of obesity. J Am Soc Nephrol 2001;12:1211–7.

26. Adolphe JL, Silver TI, Childs H, et al. Short-term obesity results in detrimental metabolic and cardiovascular changes that may not be reversed with weight loss in an obese dog model. Br J Nutr 2014;112:647–56.

27. Rocchini AP, Moorehead C, Wentz E, et al. Obesity-induced hypertension in the dog. Hypertension 1987;9(6):11164–8.

28. De Paula RB, da Silva AA, Hall JE. Aldosterone antagonism attenuates obesity-induced hypertension and glomerular hyperfiltration. Hypertension 2004;43:41–7.

29. Pinhall CS, Lopes A, Torres DB, et al. Time-course morphological and functional disorders of the kidney induced by long-term high-fat intake in female rats. Nephrol Dial Transplant 2013;28:2464–76.

30. Engli S, Bohnke J, Gorzelniak K, et al. Weight loss and the renin-angiotensin-aldosterone system. Hypertension 2005;45:356–63.

31. Pena C, Suarez L, Bautista-Castano I, et al. Effects of low-fat high-fibre diet and mitratapide on body weight reduction, blood pressure and metabolic parameters in obese dogs. J Vet Med Sci 2014;176(9):1305–8.

32. Frigolet ME, Torres N, Tovar AR. The renin-angiotensin system in adipose tissue and its metabolic consequences during obesity. J Nutr Biochem 2013;24(12): 2003–15.

33. Luo H, Wang X, Chen C. Oxidative stress causes imbalance of renal renin angiotensin system (RAS) components and hypertension in obese Zucker rats. J Am Heart Assoc 2015;4(2):102–10.

34. Grant R, Vester-Boler BM, Ridge TK, et al. Adipose tissue transcriptome changes during obesity development in female dogs. Physiol Genomics 2011;43(6): 295–307.
35. Hoenig M, Pach N, Thomaseth K, et al. Cats differ from other species in their cytokine and antioxidant enzyme response when developing obesity. Obesity (Silver Spring) 2013;21(9):E407–14.
36. Ishioka K, Omachi A, Sagawa M, et al. Canine adiponectin:cDNA structure, mRNA expression in adipose tissues and reduced plasma levels in obesity. Res Vet Sci 2006;80(2):127–32.
37. Hyung-Jin P, Sang-Eun L, Jung-Hyun O. Leptin, adiponectin and serotonin levels in lean and obese dogs. BMC Vet Res 2014;10(1):113–9.
38. Park HJ, Lee SE, Kim HB, et al. Association of obesity with serum leptin, adiponectin, and serotonin and gut microflora in beagle dogs. J Vet Intern Med 2015; 29(1):43–50.
39. Verkest KR, Rose FJ, Fleeman LM, et al. Adiposity and adiponectin in dogs: investigation of causes of discrepant results between two studies. Domest Anim Endocrinol 2011;41:35–41.
40. Hoenig M, Thomaseth K, Waldron M, et al. Insulin sensitivity, fat distribution, and adipocytokine response to different diets in lean and obese cats before and after weight loss. Am J Physiol Regul Integr Comp Physiol 2007;292(1):R227–34.
41. Ryan VH, German AJ, Wood IS, et al. Adipokine expression and secretion by canine adipocytes: stimulation of inflammatory adipokine production by LPS and TNF alpha. Pflugers Arch 2010;460(3):603–16.
42. Shibata R, Izumiya Y, Sato K, et al. Adiponectin protects against the development of systolic dysfunction following myocardial infarction. J Mol Cell Cardiol 2007;75: 1065–74.
43. Fesus G, Dubrovska G, Gorzelnaik K, et al. Adiponectin is a novel humoral vasodilator. Cardiovasc Res 2007;75:719–27.
44. Ouchi N, Ohishi M, Kihara S, et al. Association of hypoadiponectinemia with impaired vasoreactivity. Hypertension 2003;42:231–4.
45. Rocchini AP, Yang JQ, Gokee A. Hypertension and insulin resistance are not directly related in obese dogs. Hypertension 2004;43(5):1011–6.
46. Yokota T, Oritani K, Takahasi I, et al. Adiponectin, a new member of the family of soluble defence collagens, negatively regulates the growth of myelomonocytic progenitors and the functions of macrophages. Blood 2000;96:1723–32.
47. Gustafson B. Adipose tissue, inflammation and atherosclerosis. J Atheroscler Thromb 2009;17:332–41.
48. Wozniak SE, Gee LL, Wachtel MS, et al. Adipose tissue: the new endocrine organ? Dig Dis Sci 2009;54:1847–56.
49. German AJ, Hervera M, Hunter L, et al. Improvement in insulin resistance and reduction in plasma adipokines after weight loss in obese dogs. Domest Anim Endocrinol 2009;37:214–26.
50. Tvarijonaviciute A, Tecles F, Martinez-Subiela S, et al. Effect of weight loss on inflammatory biomarkers in obese dogs. Vet J 2012;193:570–2.
51. Wakshlag JJ, Struble AM, Levine CB, et al. The effects of weight loss on adipokines and markers of inflammation in dogs. Br J Nutr 2011;106:S11–4.
52. Pelosi A, Rosenstein D, Abood SK, et al. Cardiac effect of short-term experimental weight gain and loss in dogs. Vet Rec 2013;172(6):153–60.
53. Vitger AD, Stallknecht BM, Nielsen DH, et al. Integration of a physical training program in a weight loss plan for overweight pet dogs. J Am Vet Med Assoc 2016; 248(2):174–82.

54. Manens J, Ricci R, Damoiseaux C, et al. Effect of body weight loss on cardiopulmonary function assessed by 6-minute walk test and arterial blood gas analysis in obese dogs. J Vet Intern Med 2014;28:371–8.

55. Horwich TB, Fonarow GC, Hamilton MA, et al. The relationship between obesity and mortality in patients with heart failure. J Am Coll Cardiol 2001;38(3):789–95.

56. Davos CH, Doehner W, Rauchhaus M, et al. Body mass and survival in patients with chronic heart failure without cachexia: the importance of obesity. J Card Fail 2003;9(1):29–35.

57. Slupe JL, Freeman LM, Rush JE. Association of body weight and body condition with survival in dogs with heart failure. J Vet Intern Med 2008;22:561–5.

58. Finn E, Freeman LM, Rush LE, et al. The relationship between body weight, body condition and survival in cats with heart failure. J Vet Intern Med 2010;24:1369–74.

59. Curtis JP, Selter JG, Wang Y, et al. The obesity paradox. Arch Intern Med 2005;165:55–61.

60. Parameswaran K, Todd DC, Soth M. Altered respiratory physiology in obesity. Can Respir J 2006;13(4):203–10.

61. Murugan AT, Sharma G. Obesity and respiratory diseases. Chron Respir Dis 2008;5:233–42.

62. Silverstein DC, Drobatz KJ. Clinical evaluation of the respiratory tract. In: Ettinger SJ, Feldman EC, editors. Textbook of veterinary internal medicine. 7th edition. St Louis (MO): Saunders Elsevier; 2010. p. 1055–65.

63. Bach JF, Rozanski EA, Bedenice D, et al. Association of expiratory airway dysfunction with marked obesity in healthy adult dogs. Am J Vet Res 2007;68:670–5.

64. Musil KM, Petito MR, Snead ECR, et al. Blood gas values in lean and obese geriatric dogs. Abstract, ACVIM Forum Proceedings. Nashville (TN), June 4–7, 2014.

65. Manens J, Bolognin M, Bernaerts F, et al. Effects of obesity on lung function and airway reactivity in healthy dogs. Vet J 2012;193:217–21.

66. Brinson JJ, McKiernan BC. Respiratory function in obese dogs with chronic respiratory disease and their response to treatment (abstract). J Vet Intern Med 1998;12:209.

67. Garcia-Guasch L, Caro-Vadillo A, Manubens J et al. Effect of obesity on pulmonary function in cats with natural bronchial disease. ACVIM Forum Proceedings. Seattle (WA), June 12–15, 2013.

68. Champion T, Gering AP, Zacche E et al. Pulmonary function and hemogasometric evaluation of obese and overweight cats. ACVIM Forum Proceedings. Denver (CO), June 15–18, 2011.

69. Garcia-Guasch L, Caro-Vadillo A, Manubens-Grau J, et al. Pulmonary function in obese vs non-obese cats. J Feline Med Surg 2015;17(6):494–9.

70. Shore SS. Obesity and asthma: lessons from animal models. J Appl Physiol 2007;102:516–28.

71. Clercx C. Is canine eosinophilic bronchopneumopathy an asthmatic disease? ECVIM Proceedings. Munich (Germany), September 19–21, 2002.

72. Mancuso P. Obesity and respiratory infections: does excess adiposity weigh down host defence? Pulm Pharmacol Ther 2013;26(4):412–9.

73. Dhurandhar NV. Infectobesity: obesity of infectious origin. J Nutr 2001;131(10):2794S–7S.

74. Bernard A, Cohen R, Khuth ST, et al. Alteration of the leptin network in late morbid obesity induced in mice by brain infection with canine distemper. J Virol 1999;73(9):7317–27.

75. Johnson LR, Mayhew PD, Steffey MA, et al. Upper airway obstruction in Norwich terriers: 16 cases. J Vet Intern Med 2013;6(6):1409–15.
76. Hottinger H. Brachycephalic airway syndrome. Proceedings of the Western Veterinary Conference. Las Vegas (NV), February 19–23, 2006.
77. Mellema M. Non-respiratory co-morbidity of brachycephalic patients. Proceedings of International Veterinary Emergency and Critical Symposium. San Antonio (TX), September 8–12, 2012.

Obesity, Exercise and Orthopedic Disease

Christopher W. Frye, DVM[a], Justin W. Shmalberg, DVM[b], Joseph J. Wakshlag, DVM, PhD[a],*

KEYWORDS

• Obesity • Canine • Feline • Exercise • Osteoarthritis

KEY POINTS

• Obesity causes increased mechanical stress that is deleterious to the pathologic process of osteoarthritis.
• Exercise leads to higher kilocalorie intake during weight loss as well as maintenance of lean mass.
• The inflammatory milieu of obesity may lead to the worsening of osteoarthritis.
• Pathogenesis of osteoarthritis is a complex interaction between environment, mechanical stress, prior trauma, and genetics.

PATHOGENESIS OF OSTEOARTHRITIS AND INTERVERTEBRAL DISC DISEASE
Osteoarthritis

Osteoarthritis, or degenerative joint disease, is characterized by a complex progressive imbalance between cartilage production and degradation. The inciting biochemical cause of osteoarthritis remains unknown, but the condition is typically divided into primary and secondary degenerative joint disease. Primary degenerative joint disease has been hypothesized to result from repetitive loading stresses, aging, and/or a genetic predisposition, whereas secondary causes are thought to include developmental orthopedic disease, injury, and abnormal joint loading. Primary causes by definition lack a grossly identifiable structural predisposition.[1] However, this hypothesis has been challenged by some authors who interpret developmental and genetic determinants of joint and cartilage microstructure as a cause of many of the idiopathic primary cases of osteoarthritis. These may include mutations in genes encoding Type II collagen, the dominant collagen within the articular surface, in other supporting collagens such as collagens XI and IX, joint congruity, growth factors,

The authors have nothing to disclose.
[a] Department of Clinical Sciences, Cornell University College of Veterinary Medicine, Ithaca, NY 14853, USA; [b] Department of Clinical Sciences, University of Florida College of Veterinary Medicine, Gainesville, FL 32610, USA
* Corresponding author.
E-mail address: dr.joesh@gmail.com

COX-2, matrix metalloproteinase expression, TGFβ receptor or ligand, and extracellular matrix components.[1] Genes associated with hip dysplasia in dogs are linked to osteoarthritis in people,[2] and a matrix protein expressed in the ligaments around joints has been associated with hip laxity and with osteoarthritis.[3] Contributory morbidities linked to the development of secondary osteoarthritis in the dog include cranial cruciate ligament rupture, obesity, developmental orthopedic disease, and abnormal joint loading, as in the case of limb deformity or medial patellar luxation.[4–7]

The classical model of the pathogenesis of osteoarthritis focuses on the destruction of cartilage and subchondral bone, which is supported by the common histologically visible cartilage fissures and fibrillation.[8,9] The osteoarthritic joint is characterized by a loss of inherent viscoelastic properties despite chondrocyte attempts at local repair, and by changes to subchondral bone including increased bone formation and turnover.[8] Several markers of this degradative process have been identified, including interleukin (IL-1β), tumor necrosis factor alpha (TNF-α), nitric oxide, PGE_2, substance P, and matrix metalloproteinases (MMPs).[9] Early osteoarthritis secondary to medial patellar luxation is characterized by increases in the matrix metalloproteinase-2 concentration and in the expression of tartrate-resistant acid phosphatase (TRAP), a marker of collagenolytic enzyme production by synovial mononuclear cells.[4] There are no proven therapies to reverse osteoarthritis following clinical diagnosis, and therefore the focus is on preventing or slowing the process via modification of the inflammatory environment within the joint. Dogs display similar pathologic changes to osteoarthritic humans, and therefore continue to serve as a model for the condition.[6]

Osteoarthritis is commonly classified as a noninflammatory arthropathy to distinguish from autoimmune or infectious arthropathies. However, the innate immune system mediates the development of an inflammatory synovitis associated with osteoarthritis.[10] Extensive reviews of osteoarthritic synovitis have been published, but supporting evidence includes increased immune cell and toll-like receptor (TLR) activity in response to extracellular matrix components, fibronectin, plasma proteins, calcium phosphate crystals, and alarmins, which are proteins derived from damaged cells.[10] This pathophysiology has been documented in dogs; complement component 3, expressed by canine synoviocytes, is higher in dogs with stifle osteoarthritis secondary to cranial cruciate ligament insufficiency than in dogs without osteoarthritis.[11] Increased TLR-4 expression was also identified in a cruciate-deficient model of canine osteoarthritis.[12] TLRs generally recognize microbes but also respond to damage-associated molecular patterns (DAMPs), such as hyaluronan fragments, which are often elevated in the synovial fluid of osteoarthritic patients.[12] The activation of TLRs results in the production of proinflammatory chemokines, which likely increase cartilage damage.

Adiposity and obesity may affect canine osteoarthritis through several factors including increased mechanical loading, direct cell signaling, and interaction with immune cells.[7]

Intervertebral Disc Disease

Obese and overweight dogs are predisposed to intervertebral disc disease.[13] There is, however, a paucity of data regarding the interaction of disc degeneration or extrusion and obesity. Increased mechanical loading forces have been hypothesized as a primary reason for this association. Evidence in people suggests that synergism between obesity and gene mutations encoding Type IX collagen may increase risk.[14] Other clinical studies in people suggest reduced operative and nonoperative benefit to treatment in obese patients.[15] Interestingly, obesity was not a risk factor in dogs receiving a second decompressive surgery for intervertebral disc disease.[16] Obesity has also been theorized to cause challenges in clinical recovery. Obese people experience more pain than a nonobese cohort.[17] Functional mobility scores were reduced in a separate clinical study.[18] Dogs presenting to a canine referral center for neurologic rehabilitation were generally overweight, but an association to outcome was not examined.[19] Additional studies are required to understand the reasons why obese animals are predisposed to intervertebral disc disease and to determine if alterations in adipokines, inflammation, and mineralization in response to obesity play a role in the pathophysiology of the disease or in the recovery from neurologic injury.

ROLE OF ADIPOKINES IN OSTEOARTHRITIS: IS THERE A CONNECTION?

There has been a growing controversy in obesity research that revolves around the inflammation of obesity (see Robert Backus and Allison Wara's article, "Development of Obesity: Mechanisms and Physiology," in this issue). For many years, the thoughts around obesity and osteoarthritis (OA) were restricted to the mechanical effects only. Once OA has been diagnosed, undue or incongruous mechanical effects can be detrimental; however, mechanical stress alone within a joint is not sufficient to induce or further the progression of OA.[20,21] The idea of obesity having a strictly mechanical impact has been questioned, because, in people, there is a strong association between obesity and severity of hand OA despite the hand not being a mechanically stressed joint.[22,23] These findings and others surrounding hip and stifle OA in people led to further interest in the inflammatory mediators released from adipose tissue including the cytokines IL-6 and TNF-α, and the adipokines leptin, visfatin, adiponectin, and resistin (**Table 1**). The exact roles of IL-6 and TNF-α from adipose are unclear, as IL-6 and TNF-α are produced by inflamed synovial tissues as part of the pathogenesis of OA. Questions remain regarding the role of these cytokines and adipokines in the progression of the disease.

Table 1		
Inflammatory mediators released from adipose tissue		
Adipokine	**Major Actions**	**Association with OA**
Visfatin	B cell insulin secretion (NAD pathway), leukocyte adhesion, iNOS upregulation	Negative
Chemerin	Functions vary depending on cell type, insulin resistance in muscle, insulin sensitization in adipocytes, chemoattractant for immune cells	Negative
Adiponectin	Insulin sensitization (via AMPK), anti-inflammatory (decreased NF-KB), reduced gluconeogenesis, increase FFA oxidation	Positive
Leptin	Appetite regulation, increase energy expenditure, lipid oxidation, chronic inflammation	Negative
Resistin	Insulin resistance (decreased AMPK), increase IL-6, and TNF-alpha secretion, increased gluconeogenesis	Negative
IL-6	C reactive protein production, increased secretion of VLDL, inflammation, reduces adiponectin, increases leptin and chemerin	Negative
TNF-α	Increase adhesion molecules, macrophage and inflammatory cell migration, insulin resistance, NF-kB induction	Negative

Recent examination of hip and knee osteoarthritis, which are the most prevalent forms of osteoarthritis, have suggested that adipokine concentration of synovial fluid is associated with severity of osteoarthritis.[23,24] Not only synovial fluid, but also the intrapatellar fat pad, chondrocytes, and synoviocytes show varying elevations in adipokines and their receptors.[25–27] In a large meta-analysis of knee osteoarthritis, when populations were adjusted for mechanical and metabolic factors, clinical osteoarthritis was not associated with fat mass, but was associated with metabolic syndrome, suggesting the complexity goes beyond adipokines alone.[23] Leptin from adipocytes appears to be associated with increased catabolic processes in vitro. In vivo, however, leptin is associated with increased proteoglycan production. Exactly how leptin may be involved is still debated, yet the data suggest clinical signs of OA are positively associated with leptin.[28,29] The role of resistin is even less clear than that of leptin, with conflicting reports on its association with OA; however, it has been shown to increase synovitis in mouse models in higher than normal physiologic concentrations.[28,29]

The lesser known adipokines visfatin and chemerin appear to be possible culprits in the progression of OA. Visfatin is not only positively associated with obesity, it also has negative effects on cartilage and subchondral bone, inducing cytokine production and catabolic processes in articular cartilage.[30] Chemerin is a lesser known adipokine with similar catabolic effects on cartilage and an ability to induce synovitis and cytokine production at the level of the joint.[31] Similarly, the well established adipokine adiponectin is inversely associated with obesity, yet appears to be positively associated with OA in some, but not all, studies.[32–34] Adiponectin may be the most relevant adipokine, since it is one of the richest hormones in the bloodstream, and dogs may be different in their overall adipokine status than other species.[35]

This brings to light the paucity of information in dogs and cats as adipokines relate to osteoarthritis, and unlike in people, teasing away the mechanical effects may be even more difficult in a quadruped where all major affected joints are weight-bearing. Even more intriguing is rodent biology whereby certain genetic knockouts display accelerated age-related changes in cartilage or subchondral bone pathology, implicating certain genes in chronic OA.[36,37] Considering some of the subtle differences in canine and feline physiology brings to light the need to further understand how adiposity affects long-term OA from an inflammatory perspective, and how understanding local and regional adiposity in areas like the intrapatellar fat pad may provide further understanding of orthopedic diseases like cranial cruciate rupture.

ROLE OF EXERCISE IN WEIGHT LOSS

Physical activity is often recommended for the obese patient to help promote calorie expenditure, and exercise is inversely correlated with obesity in both people and pets.[38–40] Combining exercise with calorie restriction in the management of obesity reflects a contemporary standard in both human and veterinary medicine.[41–47]

Exercise alone can provide an energy deficit sufficient to cause weight loss in people consuming a diet targeting weight maintenance.[41,42,45,47] Ross and colleagues[48] demonstrated the degree of weight loss from exercise to be equivalent to diet when caloric expenditure was controlled for, yet these studies incorporate rigorous fitness programs that may not be safe considering the propensity for overheating, particularly in brachycephalic breeds. In comparison, for a 200 lb man to complete an equivalent daily exercise routine, he would have to walk briskly for 1 hour and 57 minutes daily. Differences in the intensity, type, and duration of activity or failure to control caloric intake represented confounding variables when trying to compare results from human randomized controlled trials.[48]

Unequivocally, meta-analyses conclude that physical activity alone results in less weight loss than dietary restriction; however when combined, the greatest benefits have been observed.[41,47,49]

In dogs, epidemiologic studies have demonstrated a negative relationship between obesity and activity.[38,50–53] Robertson[53] found the odds of obesity decreased with each hour of weekly activity. All of these studies, however, relied on owner surveys without further defining the amount, type, or intensity of the daily exercise, making clinical recommendations difficult. Measuring activity in dogs has also proven difficult, and many owners feel their dogs are already moderately to extremely active, demonstrating a clear bias that may undermine medical recommendations to further modify the home fitness regimen.[54]

Pedometers and accelerometers have been validated as methods to provide quantifiable data on canine activity.[38,40,44,55,56] Dogs that are less active tend to have higher body condition scores; on the other hand, animals that have finished a weight loss program did not show increased daily activity.[38,40] The success of canine fitness programs is likely multifactorial, having limitations including environment and willingness to participate. One investigation failed to find any change in canine activity despite consistently encouraging owners to lengthen walk times.[44] Additionally, dog size, device placement, and type/intensity of the exercise may influence accelerometer or pedometer data, rendering it a useful, but not an exact tool for measuring movement or energy expenditure.[44,56]

Regardless of the apparent correlations between activity and weight, few studies have described the effects of exercise on dogs when combined with caloric restriction. In a weight loss study, it was demonstrated that calorie-restricted dogs grouped as "active" based on dichotomized activity pedometer data consumed more daily calories while still achieving the same rate of weight loss as their "inactive"counterparts.[44] Similarly, dogs undergoing a mild in-hospital fitness regimen including underwater treadmill had a faster rate of weight loss over 3 months than prior reports of dogs on similar calorie-restricted meals.[43] This study had a small population size, variable limited exercise regimen, and no control group, making comparisons difficult. Mlacnik examined weight loss in a population of obese dogs with lameness by rehabilitating 1 group at home and a second group more intensely in a hospital setting. Both groups lost weight; however, with more intensive physiotherapy, a relatively greater weight reduction was noted after 60 days.[57] The exercise regimen in this study promoted 60 minutes of walking per day and electrical stimulation in the intensive therapy group; however, the amount and type of home exercise was not accurately captured over the duration of the study. Another potential bias of this study was the lack of randomization, as owners were able to choose whether to participate in hospitalized therapy. This therapy was more costly, and the choice to pursue it may have reflected commitment to the overall program including that of dietary compliance. Another study examined the effects of calorie restriction with or without exercise as it pertained to maintaining lean body mass.[58] This study was conducted over a 12-week period and showed no significant difference in weight loss between groups. The exercise group underwent 1 hour of hospitalized training 3 times weekly with underwater treadmill and land treadmill with variation in the speed and incline. Interestingly the amount and intensity of hospitalized training was greater than that previously described by Mlacnik and Chauvet, who conversely reported an increase in weight loss associated with the more active populations. The discordance between these canine studies highlights the need for a practical and stringent exercise protocol for study purposes, which is difficult to achieve in the clinical setting.

BENEFITS OF EXERCISE BEYOND WEIGHT REDUCTION

Exercise during weight loss for people includes muscular, cardiovascular, and metabolic benefits.[45,59,60] Retention of lean mass during a weight reduction program maintains a relatively higher basal metabolic rate, improves insulin sensitivity, and increases strength and function.[59–63] Lean mass in people may be further preserved by using a high-protein calorie-restricted diet, particularly a diet rich in branched-chain amino acids, which have been shown to attenuate muscle protein catabolism.[59,60]

A handful of studies have delved into the positive effects of exercise during weight loss in dogs. Dual energy x-ray absorptiometry (DEXA) has shown that lean mass was retained in exercised dogs during a dietary weight loss plan when compared with a control population.[58] As fat-free mass is considered the most metabolically active component of the basal metabolic rate, maximizing lean mass should prove beneficial to weight reduction in obese patients.[64] Alterations in the metabolic pathways in lean and fat mass have also been studied in this same subset of dogs looking for transcriptional changes within the insulin-signaling pathway.[65] Within the group of exercised dogs, muscle had higher expression of genes involved in glucose utilization and preservation of lean mass, which may reflect a positive influence on insulin signaling during the weight loss protocol.

Weight reduction may further alleviate physical disabilities and age-related orthopedic conditions. Employing calorie restriction, exercise, or a combination thereof imparts positive changes on cardiopulmonary, metabolic, and physical performance or mobility.[61] In dogs having undergone a weight loss program, cardiopulmonary health has improved based on outcomes measured by the 6-minute walk test, heart rate, and post-exercise SpO_2.[66] Beyond the 6-minute walk test, which was originally designed to assess exercise tolerance in patients with pulmonary disease, few functional tests have been established for companion animals.[67]

Physical performance or mobility, obesity status, and orthopedic disease tend to be closely related in both people and dogs. Obesity is a risk factor for OA of the knees in people, as the joint must endure greater mechanical forces through a range of physiologic movement.[68] The progression of OA is further exacerbated when joint malalignment is affecting load disbursement across the articular surface.[69–71] OA, likewise, has been positively correlated with body weight (BW) in Labrador retrievers and increases in BW may exacerbate disease-associated lameness in that population.[72,73] In a prospective randomized controlled study addressing the impact of added weight and exercise on cartilage and osteoarthritis, Beagles ran on a treadmill at 3 km per hour, 5 days per week, 75 minutes per session, over 10 years carrying 130% of their BW on back packs. No differences in gross, histopathological, or mechanical properties of stifle cartilage were observed compared with controls.[74] This study indicates that weight and exercise alone are insufficient to initiate osteoarthritis in canine stifles; however, these dogs were well conditioned, ran in a consistent fashion, had no prior orthopedic disease, and were not required to wear the weighted jackets during periods of rest, suggesting that mechanical loading is not a driving factor, and other genetic, nutritional and environmental factors are likely involved.

Validated pain and functional questionnaires and objective kinetic gait analysis have been applied to measure the outcomes of weight reduction on mobility in dogs with osteoarthritis.[75,76] A weight reduction of 8.5% to 11% in arthritic dogs was shown to alleviate orthopedic physical dysfunction, similar to the 5% reported in obese people.[75–77] Improved function and lameness scores in these canine patients, however, may not necessarily imply or result in an increase in volitional physical activity or conditioning, which is why owner and veterinary assessments are critical.

SUMMARY

Sufficient evidence exists to support that the combination of exercise with caloric restriction has the greatest efficacious impact on weight loss, body composition, and fitness health in overweight people. As of now the type, duration, and intensity of exercise has yet to be defined and may be partially dependent on the target population and diet. The preliminary canine literature hints that the addition of an exercise program may complement calorie restriction in weight loss management; however, prospective randomized controlled trials are needed with well-defined and validated outcome measures. Further examination of adipokines and their influence on OA and progression may also reveal correlations that go beyond mechanical stress, further proving that weight loss has multimodal effects that will benefit osteoarthritis. Benefits of exercise extend beyond weight loss, and include improved mobility as well as metabolic, cardiopulmonary, and muscular changes. Patient health status and owner capability may preclude certain activities, making structured rehabilitation a better alternative for some owners. Based on the current literature, a well-designed exercise program combined with an appropriate calorie-restricted diet should be recommended as the ideal treatment for overweight or obese dogs regardless of the presence of osteoarthritis so long as pain is controlled.

REFERENCES

1. Sandell LJ. Etiology of osteoarthritis: genetics and synovial joint development. Nat Rev Rheumatol 2012;8:77–89.
2. Zhou Z, Sheng X, Zhang Z, et al. Differential genetic regulation of canine hip dysplasia and osteoarthritis. PLoS One 2010;5:e13219.
3. Friedenberg SG, Zhu L, Zhang Z, et al. Evaluation of a fibrillin 2 gene haplotype associated with hip dysplasia and incipient osteoarthritis in dogs. Am J Vet Res 2011;72:530–40.
4. Alam MR, Ji JR, Kim MS, et al. Biomarkers for identifying the early phases of osteoarthritis secondary to medial patellar luxation in dogs. J Vet Sci 2011;12:273–80.
5. Szabo SD, Biery DN, Lawler DF, et al. Evaluation of a circumferential femoral head osteophyte as an early indicator of osteoarthritis characteristic of canine hip dysplasia in dogs. J Am Vet Med Assoc 2007;231:889–92.
6. Pelletier JP, Kapoor M, Fahmi H, et al. Strontium ranelate reduces the progression of experimental dog osteoarthritis by inhibiting the expression of key proteases in cartilage and of IL-1β in the synovium. Ann Rheum Dis 2013;72(2):250–7.
7. Marshall WG, Bockstahler BA, Hulse D, et al. A review of osteoarthritis and obesity: current understanding of the relationship and benefit of obesity treatment and prevention in the dog. Vet Comp Orthop Traumatol 2009;22:339–45.
8. Sharma AR, Jagga S, Lee SS, et al. Interplay between cartilage and subchondral bone contributing to pathogenesis of osteoarthritis. Int J Mol Sci 2013;14: 19805–30.
9. Sutton S, Clutterbuck A, Harris P, et al. The contribution of the synovium, synovial derived inflammatory cytokines and neuropeptides to the pathogenesis of osteoarthritis. Vet J 2009;179:10–24.

10. Sokolove J, Lepus CM. Role of inflammation in the pathogenesis of osteoarthritis: latest findings and interpretations. Ther Adv Musculoskelet Dis 2013;5:77–94.

11. Garner BC, Kuroki K, Stoker AM, et al. Expression of proteins in serum, synovial fluid, synovial membrane, and articular cartilage samples obtained from dogs with stifle joint osteoarthritis secondary to cranial cruciate ligament disease and dogs without stifle joint arthritis. Am J Vet Res 2013;74:386–94.

12. Kuroki K, Stoker AM, Sims HJ, et al. Expression of toll-like receptors 2 and 4 in stifle joint synovial tissues of dogs with or without osteoarthritis. Am J Vet Res 2010;71:750–4.

13. Packer RMA, Hendricks A, Volk HA, et al. How long and low can you go? Effect of conformation on the risk of thoracolumbar intervertebral disc extrusion in domestic dogs. PLoS One 2013;8:e69650.

14. Solovieva S, Lohiniva J, Leino-Arjas P, et al. COL9A3 gene polymorphism and obesity in intervertebral disc degeneration of the lumbar spine: evidence of gene-environment interaction. Spine 2002;27:2691–6.

15. Rihn JA, Kurd M, Hilibrand AS, et al. The influence of obesity on the outcome of treatment of lumbar disc herniation. Analysis of the Spine Patient Outcomes Research Trial (SPORT). J Bone Joint Surg Am 2013;95:1–8.

16. Dhupa S, Glickman N, Waters DJ. Reoperative neurosurgery in dogs with thoracolumbar disc disease. Vet Surg 1999;28:421–8.

17. Fanuele JC, Abdu WA, Hanscom B, et al. Association between obesity and functional status in patients with spine disease. Spine 2002;27:306–12.

18. Stenson KW, Deutsch A, Heinemann AW, et al. Obesity and inpatient rehabilitation outcomes for patients with a traumatic spinal cord injury. Arch Phys Med Rehabil 2011;92:384–90.

19. Shmalberg J, Memon MA. A retrospective analysis of 5,195 patient treatment sessions in an integrative veterinary medicine service: patient characteristics, presenting complaints, and therapeutic interventions. Vet Med Int 2015;2015: 983621.

20. Radin EL, Paul IL, Rose RM. Role of mechanical factors in pathogenesis of primary osteoarthritis. Lancet 1972;1:519–22.

21. Wildmyer MR, Utturkar GM, Leddy HA, et al. High body mass index is associated with increased diurnal strains in articular cartilage of the knee. Arthritis Rheum 2013;56:2615–22.

22. Carman WJ, Sowers M, Hawthorne VM, et al. Obesity as a risk factor for osteoarthritis of the hand and wrist: a prospective study. Am J Epidemiol 1994;139: 119–29.

23. Visser AW, de Mutsert R, le Cessie S, et al. The relative contribution of mechanical stress and systemic processes in different types of osteoarthritis: the NEO study. Ann Rheum Dis 2015;74:1842–7.

24. Gross JB, Guillaume C, Gegout-Pottie P, et al. Synovial fluid levels of adipokines in osteoarthritis: association with local factors of inflammation and cartilage maintenance. Biomed Mater Eng 2014;24:S17–25.

25. Distel E, Cadoudal T, Durant S, et al. The intrapatellar fat pad in knee osteoarthritis: an important source of interleukin-6 and its soluble receptor. Arthritis Rheum 2009;60:3374–7.

26. Ushlyama T, Chano T, Inoue K, et al. Cytokine production in the intrapatellar fat pad: another source of cytokines in knee synovial fluids. Ann Rheum Dis 2003; 62:108–12.

27. Zuo W, Wu ZH, Wu N, et al. Adiponectin receptor 1 mediates the difference in adiponectin induced prostaglandin E2 production in rheumatoid arthritis and osteoarthritis synovial fibroblast. Chin Med J 2011;124:3919–24.

28. Thijssen E, van Caam A, van der Kraan P. Obesity and osteoarthritis, more than just wear and tear: pivotal roles for inflamed adipose tissue and dyslipidaemia in obesity-induced osteoarthritis. Rheumatology 2015;54:588–600.

29. Richter M, Trzeciak T, Owecki M, et al. The role of adipocytokines in the pathogenesis of knee joint osteoarthritis. Int Orthop 2015;39:1211–7.

30. Duan Y, Hao D, Li M, et al. Increased synovial fluid visfatin is positively linked to cartilage degradation biomarkers in osteoarthritis. Rheumatol Int 2012;32: 985–90.

31. Huang K, Du G, Li L, et al. Association of chimerin levels in synovial fluid with the severity of knee osteoarthritis. Biomarkers 2012;17:16–20.

32. Yang WS, Lee WJ, Funahashi T, et al. Weight reduction increases plasma levels of an adipose derived anti-inflammatory protein adiponectin. J Clin Endocrinol Metab 2001;86:3815–9.

33. Horsawek S, Chayanupatkul M. Correlation of plasma and synovial fluid adiponectin with knee osteoarthritis severity. Arch Med Res 2010;41:593–8.

34. Lago R, Gomez R, Oteri M, et al. A new player in cartilage homeostasis: adiponectin induces nitric oxide synthase type II and pro-inflammatory cytokines in chondrocytes. Osteoarthr Cartil 2008;16:1101–9.

35. Brunson BL, Zhong Q, Clarke KJ, et al. Serum concentrations of adiponectin and characterization of adiponectin protein complexes in dogs. Am J Vet Res 2007; 68:57–62.

36. Gabay O, Sanchez C, Dvir-Ginzberg M, et al. Sirtulin 1 enzymatic activity is required for cartilage homeostasis in vivo in a mouse model. Arthritis Rheum 2013;65:159–66.

37. Gabay O, Clouse KA. Epigenetics of cartilage diseases. Joint Bone Spine 2015. [Epub ahead of print].

38. Morrison R, Reilly JJ, Penpraze V, et al. A 6-month observational study of changes in objectively measured physical activity during weight loss in dogs. J Small Anim Pract 2014;55:566–70.

39. Bauman AE, Reis RS, Sallis JF, et al. Correlates of physical activity: why are some people physically active and others not? Lancet 2012;380:258–71.

40. Chan CB, Spierenburg M, Ihle SL, et al. Use of pedometers to measure physical activity in dogs. J Am Vet Med Assoc 2005;226:126–32.

41. Jakicic JM, Otto AD. Physical activity considerations for the treatment and prevention of obesity. Am J Clin Nutr 2005;82:226–9.

42. Roudebush P, Schoenherr WD, Delaney SJ. An evidence-based review of the use of therapeutic foods, owner education, exercise, and drugs for the management of obese and overweight pets. J Am Vet Med Assoc 2008;232:717–23.

43. Chauvet A, Laclair J, Elliott DA, et al. Incorporation of exercise, using an underwater treadmill, and active client education into a weight management program for obese dogs. Can Vet J 2011;52:491–6.

44. Wakshlag JJ, Struble AM, Warren BS, et al. Evaluation of dietary energy intake and physical activity in dogs undergoing a controlled weight-loss program. J Am Vet Med Assoc 2012;240:413–9.

45. Ross R, Dagnone D, Jones P, et al. Reduction in obesity and related comorbid conditions after diet-induced weight loss or exercise-induced weight loss in men. Ann Intern Med 2000;133:92.

46. Lee S, Kuk JL, Davidson LE, et al. Role of exercise in reducing the risk of diabetes and obesity exercise without weight loss is an effective strategy for obesity reduction in obese individuals with and without Type 2 diabetes. J Appl Physiol (1985) 2005;6:1220–5.

47. Catenacci VA, Wyatt H. The role of physical activity in producing and maintaining weight loss. Nat Clin Pract Endocrinol Metab 2015;3:518–29.

48. Ross R, Jansenn J, Dawson J, et al. Exercise-induced reduction in obesity and insulin resistance in women: a randomized controlled trial. Obes Res 2004;12: 789–98.

49. Miller WC, Koceja DM, Hamilton EJ. A meta-analysis of the past 25 years of weight loss research using diet, exercise or diet plus exercise intervention. Int J Obes Relat Metab Disord 1997;21:941–7.

50. Courcier EA, Thomson RM, Mellor DJ, et al. An epidemiological study of environmental factors associated with canine obesity. J Small Anim Pract 2010;51:362–7.

51. Mao J, Xia Z, Chen J, et al. Prevalence and risk factors for canine obesity surveyed in veterinary practices in Beijing, China. Prev Vet Med 2013;112:438–42.

52. Raffan E, Smith SP, O'Rahilly S, et al. Development, factor structure and application of the Dog Obesity Risk and Appetite (DORA) questionnaire. PeerJ 2015;3: e1278.

53. Robertson ID. The association of exercise, diet and other factors with owner-perceived obesity in privately owned dogs from metropolitan Perth, WA. Prev Vet Med 2003;58:75–83.

54. Slater M, Robinson L, Zoran D, et al. Diet and exercise patterns in pet dogs. J Am Vet Med Assoc 1995;2:186–90.

55. Yam PS, Penpraze V, Young D, et al. Validity, practical utility and reliability of Actigraph accelerometry for the measurement of habitual physical activity in dogs. J Small Anim Pract 2011;52:86–91.

56. Preston T, Baltzer W, Trost S. Accelerometer validity and placement for detection of changes in physical activity in dogs under controlled conditions on a treadmill. Res Vet Sci 2012;93:412–6.

57. Mlacnik E, Bockstahler BA, Müller M, et al. Effects of caloric restriction and a moderate or intense physiotherapy program for treatment of lameness in overweight dogs with osteoarthritis. J Am Vet Med Assoc 2006;229:1756–60.

58. Vitger AD, Stallknecht BM, Nielsen DH, et al. Integration of a physical activity in a Weight Loss Plan for Overweight Pet Dogs. J Am Vet Med Assoc 2016;248: 174–82.

59. Dudgeon WD, Kelley EP, Scheett TP. In a single-blind, matched group design: branched-chain amino acid supplementation and resistance training maintains lean body mass during a caloric restricted diet. J Int Soc Sports Nutr 2016;13:1.

60. Verreijen AM, de Wilde J, Engberink MF, et al. A high whey protein, leucine enriched supplement preserves muscle mass during intentional weight loss in obese older adults: a double blind randomized controlled trial. Clin Nutr 2013; 32:S3.

61. Villareal DT, Chode S, Parimi N, et al. Weight loss, exercise, or both and physical function in obese older adults. N Engl J Med 2011;364:1218–29.

62. Votruba SB, Horvitz MA, Schoeller DA. The role of exercise in the treatment of obesity. Nutrition 2000;16:179–88.

63. Curioni CC, Lourenço PM. Long-term weight loss after diet and exercise: a systematic review. Int J Obes 2005;29:1168–74.

64. Larsson C, Vitger A, Jensen RB, et al. Evaluation of the oral 13C-bicarbonate technique for measurements of energy expenditure in dogs before and after body weight reduction. Acta Vet Scand 2014;56:1–7.
65. Herrera Uribe J, Vitger AD, Ritz C, et al. Physical training and weight loss in dogs lead to transcriptional changes in genes involved in the glucose-transport pathway in muscle and adipose tissues. Vet J 2015;208:22–7.
66. Manens J, Ricci R, Damoiseaux C, et al. Effect of body weight loss on cardiopulmonary function assessed by 6-minute walk test and arterial blood gas analysis in obese dogs. J Vet Intern Med 2014;28:371–8.
67. Swimmer RA, Rozanski E. Evaluation of the 6-minute walk test in pet dogs. J Vet Intern Med 2011;25:405–6.
68. Zheng H, Chen C. Body mass index and risk of knee osteoarthritis: systematic review and meta-analysis of prospective studies. BMJ Open 2015;5:e007568.
69. Tanamas S, Hanna FS, Cicuttini FM, et al. Does knee malalignment increase the risk of development and progression of knee osteoarthritis? A systematic review. Arthritis Rheum 2009;61:459–67.
70. Felson DT, Goggins J, Niu J, et al. The effect of body weight on progression of knee osteoarthritis is dependent on alignment. Arthritis Rheum 2004;50:3904–9.
71. Brouwer GM, Van Tol AW, Bergink AP, et al. Association between valgus and varus alignment and the development and progression of radiographic osteoarthritis of the knee. Arthritis Rheum 2007;56:1204–11.
72. Kealy RD, Lawler DF, Ballam JM, et al. Evaluation of the effect of limited food consumption on radiographic evidence of osteoarthritis in dogs. J Am Vet Med Assoc 2000;217:1678–80.
73. Moreau M, Troncy A, Bichot S, et al. Influence of changes in body weight on peak vertical force in osteoarthritic dogs: a possible bias in study outcome. Vet Surg 2010;39:43–7.
74. Newton PM, Mow VC, Gardner TR, et al. The effect of lifelong exercise on canine articular cartilage. Am J Sports Med 1997;25:282–7.
75. Impellizeri JA, Tetrick MA, Muir P. Effect of weight reduction on clinical signs of lameness in dogs with hip osteoarthritis. J Am Vet Med Assoc 2000;216(7):1089–91.
76. Marshall WG, Hazewinkel HA, Mullen D, et al. The effect of weight loss on lameness in obese dogs with osteoarthritis. Vet Res Commun 2010;34:241–53.
77. Christensen R, Bartels EM, Astrup A, et al. Effect of weight reduction in obese patients diagnosed with knee osteoarthritis: a systematic review and meta-analysis. Ann Rheum Dis 2006;66(4):433–9.

Other Risks/Possible Benefits of Obesity

Lisa P. Weeth, DVM, MRCVS[a,b,*]

KEYWORDS

- Obesity • Hyperlipidemia • Adipokines • Renal • Quality of life

KEY POINTS

- Obese individuals have changes to the intestinal microbiome that may influence overall health and well-being.
- Adipocytes produce cytokines that may act to promote neoplastic changes to other cell lines.
- Obesity is considered a significant risk factor in development of chronic renal failure in people; in dogs, obesity can lead to altered renal function and histologic changes to renal architecture.
- Obese and overweight dogs have lower quality of life assessments and potentially shorter lifespan relative to lean dogs.

INTRODUCTION

Before the discovery of leptin, any adverse effects of obesity were attributed to mechanical stress on cardiovascular and musculoskeletal systems, but now it is known that adipocytes secrete hormones and cytokines that can have long-term adverse effects on health and wellness[1] (see Melissa Clark and Margarethe Hoenig's article, "Metabolic Effects of Obesity and Its Interaction with Endocrine Diseases," in this issue). Obesity results in a chronic inflammatory condition[2] that can predispose the individual to development of diabetes mellitus, hypertension, and nonhypertensive renal disease.[3] Obese people, for example, have a higher risk of developing atopic dermatitis,[4] are at an increased risk of developing certain cancers,[5–7] and have an increased risk of mortality from other diseases.[8]

Obesity is defined as the accumulation of excess adiposity and is one of the most common forms of malnutrition seen in otherwise well cared for domestic dogs and cats. Animals that are more than 20% over their ideal weight are considered obese[9] and published literature on canine and feline obesity prevalence indicate that between 34% and 63% of the dog and cat populations are either overweight or obese.[10–15]

The author has nothing to disclose.
[a] Weeth Nutrition Services, 25 Chester Street, Edinburgh EH3 7EN, UK; [b] Clinical Nutrition Department, Telemedicine Services, Gulf Coast Veterinary Specialists, 1111 West Loop South, Houston, TX 77027, USA
* Weeth Nutrition Services, 25 Chester Street, Edinburgh EH3 7EN, UK.
E-mail address: weethnutrition@gmail.com

Excess adiposity in dogs and cats has a significant impact on the development of degenerative orthopedic disease,[16] insulin-resistance,[17] and diabetes mellitus.[11,12] It also impairs pulmonary function[18] and increases the risk of death from heat stroke in dogs.[19] Obese dogs and cats also have a higher prevalence of nonallergic skin disease[11,12,20,21] and lower urinary tract disease signs[11,12,22] compared with their lean cohorts (**Box 1**).

OBESITY AS A CHRONIC INFLAMMATORY CONDITION

Leptin, resistin, adiponectin, vascular endothelial growth factor, interleukin (IL)-6, and tumor necrosis factor (TNF)-α are among the adipose-derived cytokines (adipokines) and inflammatory mediators secreted by adipocytes. The elevated plasma concentrations of compounds, such as leptin, resistin, IL-6, and TNF-α, have been well documented in people[2] and have also been seen in obese dogs and cats.[23–32] Leptin is positively associated with body fat mass and increases or decreases with adiposity. Under normal homeostatic conditions leptin receptors on the hypothalamus provide feedback to the brain to control food intake, and subsequently body weight, within a specific metabolic range.[1] Obese dogs and cats have higher serum levels of leptin than lean counterparts.[23–32] Prolonged elevations in these adipokines either independently or in concert may set the stage for future metabolic derangement by inducing peripheral insulin resistance, propagating pain signaling, or altering circulating levels of serum lipids.[33]

Studies in obese dogs have also found higher levels of cortisol[28,29] and higher circulating levels of IL-6, TNF-α, and monocyte chemoattractant protein 1 concentrations relative to lean dogs.[26,27] IL-6 and TNF-α are proinflammatory mediators and are considered nonspecific markers of chronic inflammation; monocyte chemoattractant protein 1 promotes migration of inflammatory cells into a given area. This degree of constant low-grade inflammation has been theorized to result in altered immune function, but studies to this effect in dogs and cats have been limited. Obese puppies may have an increased risk of fatal complications from distemper virus.[34] Conversely, modest calorie restriction and maintenance of a lean body condition score (BCS) may slow age-related decline in immune cell function in dogs.[35] Dogs that maintained

Box 1		
Health risks of obesity in dogs and cats		
Known Heath Risks of Obesity	**Species (Dog/Cat)**	**Reference**
Increased risk/worsening of orthopedic disease	Dog/cat	16,88,89
Decreased overall activity	Dog	82,83
Increased risk of insulin resistance, diabetes mellitus	Dog/cat	11,12,17
Pulmonary dysfunction	Dog/cat	18
Increased risk of death from heat stroke	Dog	19
Increased risk nonallergic skin disease	Dog/cat	11,12,20,21
Increased risk lower urinary tract disease signs	Dog/cat	11,12,22
Altered intestinal flora	Dog/cat	29,45,46
Altered renal function, histologic changes to renal architecture	Dog	77–79
Hyperlipidemia	Dog/cat	26,28,42,49,50
Hepatic lipid accumulation	Dog/cat	53,56–58
Increased risk certain cancers	Dog	63–65,67,68
Decreased quality of life parameters (owner assessment)	Dog	86–89
Decreased life span	Dog	16,35

a lean BCS (average BCS, 4.6/9) in this study had less of an age-related decline in lymphoproliferative response to mitogens and less of an age-related decline in total lymphocyte counts, T-cell populations, and CD-4 and CD-8 cell lines compared with dogs that maintained an overweight BCS (average BCS, 6.7/9).[35]

The inflammatory mediators IL-6 and TNF-α do not seem to be altered by obesity in cats.[33] Experimentally induced short-term obesity in cats also does not seem to change lymphocyte cell counts or mitogen response.[36] Controlled long-term obesity studies similar to those performed in dogs evaluating the immunologic effect of lifetime overweightedness or obesity in cats has not been performed to date.

Adiponectin is secreted by adipocytes, but unlike leptin, is inversely related to body fat mass.[37] Adiponectin stimulates fatty acid oxidation in hepatic cells and sensitizes cell to insulin and is considered beneficial for overall glucose and fatty acid homeostasis. Decreased serum adiponectin concentrations are also found in obese cats,[33,38] but reports in obese dogs are inconsistent. Some studies have shown decreased levels of adiponectin in obese dogs,[25,28,29,39,40] whereas others[30,41] found normal adiponectin levels in obese relative to lean dogs. The mechanism behind obesity's influence on adiponectin secretion is unclear and may be related to inhibitory effects of inflammatory mediators, such as IL-6 and TNF-α.[37]

GASTROINTESTINAL HEALTH

Obese dogs also have lower serotonin (5-hydroxytryptamine [5HT]) levels.[28] Enterochromaffin cells in the intestinal epithelium release 5HT in response to food in the lumen. Under normal dietary situations circulating concentrations of this neurotransmitter increase after a meal, but high-fat meals and obesity seem to reduce enterochromaffin cell numbers resulting in lower 5HT concentrations overall.[42] Lower 5HT levels slow colonic transit time and have been proposed as a contributing factor to obesity-induced constipation in people.[43] Obese cats have a higher prevalence of constipation,[12] although 5HT concentrations in obese cats and any potential association with constipation have not been published to date.

The slower gastrointestinal transit time may allow for greater fermentation of undigested carbohydrates and fats potentially altering the colonic microbiome. Obese dogs and cats have a significantly different microbiome than lean individuals[29,44] with a lower diversity of gut bacterial species.[29] Park and colleagues[29] found that lean dogs had predominantly gram-positive Firmicutes, such as *Lactobacillus*, whereas obese dogs had a higher prevalence of gram-negative strains, such as *Pseudomonas*. Increased numbers of clostridial bacteria have also been found in obese dogs,[45] although this was not found in all studies.[29,44] Large populations of gram-negative bacteria can increase intestinal lipopolysaccharide levels, which has been associated with chronic gastrointestinal inflammation in experimental mouse models.[46] Even in the absence of a local adverse reaction to intestinal microflora, higher concentrations of acetate and butyrate have also been found within the intestinal lumen of obese individuals[47] indicating that bacterial fermentation may result in greater energy extraction from the diet. It is not clear if obesity induces intestinal bacterial dysbiosis or if dysbiosis influences obesity, but this is a growing area of research.

HYPERLIPIDEMIA, PANCREATIC, AND LIVER DYSFUNCTION

Obesity is one of the more common causes of hyperlipidemia in dogs and cats.[26,28,38,48–50] In one study, even moderate obesity (BCS, 7–7.5/9) resulted in higher serum triglyceride concentrations relative to lean (BCS, 4–5/9) dogs.[28] Obese cats also have higher cholesterol and triglyceride concentrations[38,49] with specific increases in the circulating very-low-density lipoprotein concentration.[50] Increased concentrations of canine pancreatic lipase immunoreactivity and concurrent hypertriglyceridemia have also been demonstrated in overweight and obese dogs.[48] Hyperlipidemia is a known trigger for acute necrotizing pancreatitis in humans[51] and in rodent models[52] and has been theorized as a risk factor for pancreatitis in dogs.[53] The risk of acute fatal pancreatitis increases with increasing adiposity in dogs,[11,54] although whether this was a causative or correlated in these retrospective studies was not clear.

Hyperlipidemia has also been associated with development of gallbladder mucoceles in dogs.[55] Increased hepatocellular triglycerides and cholesterol occurs with hyperlipidemia in dogs resulting in overt hepatic lipidosis[53] and vacuolar hepatopathy.[56] Cats accumulate fat within the liver after weight gain and development of obesity[57] and are at an increased risk of developing clinically significant hepatic lipidosis during periods of starvation and extreme weight loss. Elevated alanine aminotransferase, alkaline phosphatase, and γ-glutamyltransferase levels have also been demonstrated in obese dogs and are correlated with hypercholesterolemia.[58] However, Yamka and colleagues[59] found only elevations in alkaline phosphatase, without changes in alanine aminotransferase or γ-glutamyltransferase in obese dogs, whereas Pena and colleagues[60] found no significant difference in alanine aminotransferase concentrations between lean and overweight/obese dogs (although obese [ie, BCS >7/9] dogs were not evaluated separately from overweight dogs [ie, BCS, 6/9] and alkaline phosphatase and γ-glutamyltransferase levels were not reported).

OBESITY AND CANCER RISK

Elevated levels of leptin, resistin, IL-6, and TNF-α inhibit normal apoptotic mechanisms and promote angiogenesis,[33] which may serve as cancer promoters in vivo. Leptin specifically is an in vitro promoter of mammary tumors[61] and hepatocellular carcinomas[62] in humans; to date, this specific relationship between adipokines and tumorigenesis has not been documented in dogs and cats.

Obese dogs and cats have an increased prevalence of benign and malignant neoplasms overall.[11,12] There are a limited number of retrospective studies that have evaluated the association of specific cancer types and obesity.[63–68] Glickman and colleagues[63] collected owner-reported obesity status 1-year before diagnosis of transitional cell carcinoma of the urinary bladder of dogs, finding that there was an increased prevalence of obesity in affected dogs. Sonnenschein and colleagues[64] and Perez Alenza and colleagues[65] found that there was a positive correlation between mammary tumor development and owner-reported obesity, but not between body weight as recorded in the medical record compared with the breed standard for the individual. Philibert and colleagues[66] only used documented body weight versus breed standard and also found no association with obesity and mammary tumor development. More recent studies have found positive associations between obesity and mammary cancer development when clinical measures of obesity (ie, BCS) are used. A retrospective study of dogs presenting to a referral veterinary teaching hospital showed a higher prevalence of overweightedness and obesity (BCS $\geq$6/9) in dogs with mammary cancers,[69] although this result did not reach statistical significance. Lim and colleagues[67,68] found that female dogs with a BCS greater than 7 develop mammary cancer at an earlier age than lean dogs and had worse histologic prognostic indicators.

Mortality data from a long-term prospective study on calorie restriction in Labrador retrievers showed an equal distribution of cancers among control dogs (mean BCS,

6.7/9) and restricted-fed dogs (mean BCS, 4.6/9).[70] The variety of cancer types reported, limited sample size, and the avoidance of overt obesity in control dogs make direct conclusions about obesity and cancer development in that study difficult. Interestingly, for the 11 dogs that developed fatal cancers, the mean age of death for control-fed dogs was 9.7 years (N = 6), whereas the mean age at death for five restricted-fed dogs was 11.6 years (N = 5).[35] A BCS survey of canine patients with cancer found that out of 100 dogs presenting to the oncology service at a veterinary referral teaching hospital, 26 dogs were considered overweight and 29 dogs were considered obese using a nine-point BCS scale.[71] This investigation was focused on cancer cachexia and, as such, associations between obesity and cancer prevalence cannot be made based on the study design and sample size.[71]

EFFECTS ON RENAL FUNCTION AND HISTOLOGY

Obesity is considered a significant risk factor in development of chronic renal failure in people.[72,73] Chronically obese individuals are at a high risk of developing glomerularsclerosis independent of diabetes mellitus or systemic hypertension[74] and reducing fat mass can improve renal parameters.[75,76] In dogs, obesity is associated with mild hypertension but this finding is minor and does not typically warrant medical intervention, although even mild hypertension can result in a concomitant increase in heart rate and an increased sodium resorption from the renal tubules resulting in glomerular hyperfiltration, renal hypertension, and insidious damage to the renal parenchyma.[77]

Experimentally induced obesity in dogs increases mean arterial pressure and plasma renin activity, which alters renal function and causes histologic changes to renal architecture. Expansion of Bowman capsule, cell proliferation in glomeruli, thickening of glomerular and tubular basement membrane, and increased mesangial matrix can be seen.[78] Obese dogs also have increased levels of biomarkers of renal injury (homocysteine, cystatin, and clusterin), which improve after weight loss,[79] and glomerular leakage caused by changes to Bowman capsule has been proposed to result in pathologic proteinuria. Mildly increased urine protein to creatinine ratios were seen in one obese population of dogs,[79] which resolved with weight loss. Another study showed no significant difference in median urine protein to creatinine ratio values between lean and overweight/obese dogs.[80] In humans, the magnitude of proteinuria is positively correlated with degree of obesity[81] and by grouping all overweight and obese dogs together Tefft and colleagues[80] may have masked this effect.

EFFECTS ON QUALITY OF LIFE AND LONGEVITY

Overweight and obese dogs have lower activity levels compared with lean dogs[82,83]; whether this was caused by underlying comorbidities (eg, osteoarthritis), a direct effect of excess body weight, an indirect effect of adipokine production, or another mechanism is not clear. Obese people who lost weight report improved quality of life parameters especially in physical fitness and vitality assessments.[84,85] Obese and overweight dogs that lost at least 15% of their body weight had improvement in owner assessments of quality of life as measured by indicators of vitality, activity, and emotional well-being.[86–89] Obese dogs with osteoarthritis also had reduction in disease severity scores and increased physical activity and mental alertness when they lost weight.[88,89]

Calorie restriction, rather than avoidance of obesity, has been shown to increase lifespan in rodent and primate models[90] and dogs.[16] In a long-term study of Labrador retrievers fed a controlled calorie intake found that dogs fed to maintain a lean body condition (mean BCS, 4.6/9) lived an average of 1.8 years longer than overweight dogs (mean BCS, 6.7/9)[16]; the median lifespan for control-fed dogs was 11.2 years, compared with 13 years for the restricted-fed dogs. Restricted-fed dogs in that study not only lived longer than the control-fed dogs, they had a delay in treatment of chronic conditions by 2.1 years; the median age of treatment of chronic conditions in the restricted-fed group was 12.0 years (range, 4.0–14.4 years) and 9.9 years (range, 4.6–12.9 years) in the overweight control-fed group.

OBESITY PARADOX?

In people, increased body mass index is associated with lower risk of mortality from congestive heart failure and a lower risk of in-hospital mortality compared with normal weight or underweight individuals.[91–93] This seemingly protective effect of obesity is termed the obesity paradox. Similar to people, overweight and obese dogs and cats with heart failure may have improved survival times over lean animals. Positive correlations have been seen between survival times and increasing BCS in dogs and cats with heart failure, although these results did not reach statistical significance.[94,95] Dogs with renal disease that were either overweight (BCS, 7–9/9) or had what was considered a more ideal body weight (BCS, 4–6/9) at the time of diagnosis also had improved survival times compared with dogs that were considered underweight (BCS, 1–3/9), but BCS was also significantly correlated with disease severity in that survey.[96]

The obesity paradox is theorized to be related to protective neuroendocrine factors secreted from adipose tissue, a lack of cachexia, and/or a protective effect of excess body weight. Weight gain and development of obesity is the result of increases in lean and fat mass, with approximately 75% of the added weight coming from expansion of adipocytes and the remaining 25% from lean body mass accretion.[97] Therefore it is possible that obese animals have greater lean body mass reserves during periods of poor food intake and it is the avoidance of cachexia, rather than a beneficial effect of obesity, that improves outcomes in these patients.

SUMMARY

Obesity is not a cosmetic or social issue; it is an animal health issue. The metabolic effects of obesity on insulin resistance and development of hyperlipidemia and the mechanical stress excess weight places on the musculoskeletal system are fairly well established in the literature. Additional health risks from obesity, such as fatty accumulation in the liver, intestinal bacterial dysbiosis, and changes to renal architecture, are less well understood, but have been demonstrated to occur clinically in obese animals nonetheless and may lead to deleterious long-term health effects. Keeping dogs and cats lean not only lowers their risk for development of certain diseases, but can lead to a longer and better quality of life.

REFERENCES

1. Signore AP, Zhang F, Weng Z, et al. Leptin neuroprotection in the CNS: mechanism and therapeutic potential. J Neurochem 2008;106:1977–99.

2. Cottam DR, Mattar SG, Barinas-Mitchell E, et al. The chronic inflammatory hypothesis for the morbidity associated with morbid obesity: implications and effects of weight loss. Obes Surg 2004;14(5):589–600.

3. Gabbay E, Slotki I, Shavit L. Weighing the evidence: obesity, metabolic syndrome, and the risk of chronic kidney disease. BMC Nephrol 2015;16:133–6.

4. Zhang A, Silverberg JI. Association of atopic dermatitis with being overweight and obese: a systematic review and metaanalysis. J Am Acad Dermatol 2015; 72:606–16.

5. Wei EK, Giovannucci E, Wu K, et al. Comparison of risk factors for colon and rectal cancer. Int J Cancer 2004;108:433–42.

6. van den Brandt PA, Spiegelman D, Yaun SS, et al. Pooled analysis of prospective cohort studies on height, weight, and breast cancer risk. Am J Epidemiol 2000; 152:514–27.

7. Takeda T, Sakata M, Isobe A, et al. Relationship between metabolic syndrome and uterine leiomyomas: a case-control study. Gynecol Obstet Invest 2008;66: 14–7.

8. Calle EE, Thun MJ. Obesity and cancer. Oncogene 2004;23:6365–78.

9. Mawby DI, Bartges JW, d'Avignon A, et al. Comparison of various methods for estimating body fat in dogs. J Am Anim Hosp Assoc 2004;40:109–14.

10. O'Neill DG, Church DB, McGreevy PD, et al. Prevalence of disorders recorded in cats attending primary-care veterinary practices in England. Vet J 2014;202: 286–91.

11. Lund EM, Armstrong PJ, Kirk CA, et al. Prevalence and risk factors for obesity in adult dogs from private US veterinary practices. Int J Appl Res Vet Med 2006;4: 177–86.

12. Lund EM, Armstrong PJ, Kirk CA, et al. Prevalence and risk factors for obesity in adult cats from private US veterinary practices. Int J Appl Res Vet Med 2005;3: 88–96.

13. Courcier EA, Mellor DJ, Pendlebury E, et al. An investigation into the epidemiology of feline obesity in Great Britain: results of a cross-sectional study of 47 companion animal practices. Vet Rec 2012;171:560.

14. Courcier EA, O'Higgins R, Mellor DJ, et al. Prevalence and risk factors for feline obesity in a first opinion practice in Glasgow, Scotland. J Feline Med Surg 2010; 12:746–53.

15. Cave NJ, Allan FJ, Schokkenbroek SL, et al. A cross-sectional study to compare changes in the prevalence and risk factors for feline obesity between 1993 and 2007 in New Zealand. Prev Vet Med 2012;107:121–33.

16. Kealy RD, Lawler DF, Ballam JM, et al. Effects of diet restriction on life span and age-related changes in dogs. J Am Vet Med Assoc 2002;220:1315–20.

17. Mattheeuws D, Rottiers R, Kaneko JJ, et al. Diabetes mellitus in dogs: relationship of obesity to glucose tolerance and insulin response. Am J Vet Res 1984;45: 98–103.

18. Garcia-Guasch L, Caro-Vadilla A, Manubeus-Grau J, et al. Pulmonary function in obese vs non-obese cats. J Feline Med Surg 2015;17:494–9.

19. Bruchim Y, Klement E, Saragusty J, et al. Heat stroke in dogs: a retrospective study of 54 cases (1999–2004) and analysis of risk factors for death. J Vet Intern Med 2006;20:38–46.

20. Scarlett JM, Donoghue S. Associations between body condition and disease in cats. J Am Vet Med Assoc 1998;212:1725–31.

21. Mason E. Obesity in pet dogs. Vet Rec 1970;86:612–6.

22. Lekcharoensuk C, Lulich JP, Osborne CA, et al. Association between patient-related factors and risk of calcium oxalate and magnesium ammonium phosphate urolithiasis in cats. J Am Vet Med Assoc 2000;217:520–5.

23. Gayet C, Bailhache E, Dumon H, et al. Insulin resistance and changes in plasma concentration of TNFα, IGF1, and NEFA in dogs during weight gain and obesity. J Anim Physiol Anim Nutr (Berl) 2004;88:157–65.

24. Martin LJM, Siliart B, Dumon HJW, et al. Hormonal disturbances associated with obesity in dogs. J Anim Physiol Anim Nutr (Berl) 2006;90:355–60.

25. Ishioka K, Soliman MM, Sagawa M, et al. Experimental and clinical studies on plasma leptin in obese dogs. J Vet Med Sci 2002;64:349–53.

26. Jeusette IC, Lhoest ET, Istasse LP, et al. Influence of obesity on plasma lipid and lipoprotein concentrations in dogs. Am J Vet Res 2005;66:81–6.

27. Frank L, Mann S, Levine CB, et al. Increasing body condition score is positively associated interleukin-6 and monocyte chemoattractant protein-1 in Labrador retrievers. Vet Immunol Immunopathol 2015;167:104–9.

28. Park HJ, Lee SE, Oh JH, et al. Leptin, adiponectin and serotonin levels in lean and obese dogs. BMC Vet Res 2014;10:113.

29. Park HJ, Lee SE, Kim HB, et al. Association of obesity with serum leptin, adiponectin, and serotonin and gut microflora in Beagle dogs. J Vet Intern Med 2015; 29:43–50.

30. Wakshlag JJ, Struble AM, Levine CB, et al. The effects of weight loss on adipokines and markers of inflammation in dogs. Br J Nutr 2011;106:S11–4.

31. Van de Velde H, Janssens GPJ, de Rooster H, et al. The cat as a model for human obesity: insights into depot-specific inflammation associated with feline obesity. Br J Nutr 2013;110:1326–35.

32. Hoenig M, Pach N, Thomaseth K, et al. Cats differ from other species in their cytokine and antioxidant enzyme response when developing obesity. Obesity 2013; 21:E407–14.

33. Zou C, Shao J. Role of adipocytokines in obesity-associated insulin resistance. J Nutr Biochem 2008;19:277–86.

34. Newberne PM. Overnutrition on resistance of dogs to distemper virus. Fed Proc 1966;25:1701–10.

35. Lawler DF, Larson BT, Ballam JM, et al. Diet restriction and ageing in the dog: major observations over two decades. Br J Nutr 2008;99:793–805.

36. Jaso-Friedmann L, Leary JH 3rd, Praveen K, et al. The effects of obesity and fatty acids on the feline immune system. Vet Immunol Immunopathol 2008;122: 146–52.

37. Chakraborti CK. Role of adiponectin and some other factors linking type 2 diabetes mellitus and obesity. World J Diabetes 2015;6:1296–308.

38. Muranaka S, Mori N, Hatano Y, et al. Obesity induced changes to plasma adiponectin concentration and cholesterol lipoprotein composition profile in cats. Res Vet Sci 2011;91:358–61.

39. Eirmann LA, Freeman LM, Laflamme DP, et al. Comparison of adipokine concentrations and markers of inflammation in obese versus lean dogs. Int J Appl Res Vet Med 2009;7:196–205.

40. Tvarijonaviciute A, Ceron JJ, Shelley L, et al. Obesity-related metabolic dysfunction in dogs: a comparison with human metabolic syndrome. BMC Vet Res 2012; 8:147.

41. German AJ, Hervera M, Hunter L, et al. Improvement in insulin resistance and reduction in plasma inflammatory adipokines after weight loss in obese dogs. Domest Anim Endocrinol 2009;37:214–26.

42. Bertrand RL, Senadheera S, Tanoto A, et al. Serotonin availability in rat colon is reduced during a Western diet model of obesity. Am J Physiol Gastrointest Liver Physiol 2012;303:G424–34.

43. Mushref MA, Srinivasan S. Effect of high fat-diet and obesity on gastrointestinal motility. Ann Transl Med 2013;1:14.

44. Keiler IN, Molbak L, Hansen LL, et al. Overweight and the feline gut microbiome - a pilot study. J Anim Physiol Anim Nutr (Berl) 2015. http://dx.doi.org/10.1111/jpn. 12409.

45. Handl S, German AJ, Holden SL, et al. Faecal microbiota in lean and obese dogs. FEMS Microbiol Ecol 2013;84:332–43.

46. Im E, Rieger FM, Pothoulakis C, et al. Elevated lipopolysaccaride in the colon evokes intestinal inflammation aggravated in immune-impaired mice. Am J Physiol Gastrointest Liver Physiol 2012;303:G490–7.

47. Turnbaugh PJ, Ley RE, Mahowald MA, et al. An obesity-associated gut microbiome with increased capacity for energy harvest. Nature 2006;444:1027–31.

48. Verkest KR, Fleeman LM, Morton JM, et al. Association of postprandial serum triglyceride concentration and serum canine pancreatic lipase immunoreactivity in overweight and obese dogs. J Vet Intern Med 2012;26:46–53.

49. Mori N, Okada Y, Tsuchida N, et al. Preliminary analysis of modified low-density lipoprotein in serum of healthy and obese dogs and cats. Front Vet Sci 2015;2:34.

50. Hoenig M, Wilkins C, Holson JC, et al. Effects of obesity on lipid profiles in neutered male and female cats. Am J Vet Res 2003;64:299–303.

51. Kota SK, Kota SK, Jannula S, et al. Hypertriglyceridemia-induced recurrent acute pancreatitis: a case-based review. Indian J Endocrinol Metab 2012;16:141–5.

52. Hofbauer B, Friess H, Weber A, et al. Hyperlipaemia intensifies the course of acute oedematous and acute necrotising pancreatitis in the rat. Gut 1996;38: 753–8.

53. Xenoulis PG, Steiner JM. Canine hyperlipidaemia. J Small Anim Pract 2015;56: 595–605.

54. Hess RS, Kass PH, Shofer FS, et al. Evaluation of risk factors for fatal acute pancreatitis in dogs. J Am Vet Med Assoc 1999;214:46–51.

55. Kutsunai M, Kanemoto H, Fukushima K, et al. The association between gall bladder mucoceles and hyperlipidaemia in dogs: a retrospective case control study. Vet J 2014;199:76–9.

56. Sandoe P, Palmer C, Corr S, et al. Canine and feline obesity: a one health perspective. Vet Rec 2014;175:610–4.

57. Nicoll RG, Jackson MW, Knipp BS, et al. Quantitative ultrasonography of the liver in cats during obesity induction and dietary restriction. Res Vet Sci 1998;64:1–6.

58. Tribuddharatana T, Kongpiromchean Y, Sribhen K, et al. Biochemical alterations and their relationships with the metabolic syndrome components in canine obesity. Kasetsart J (Nat Sci) 2011;45:622–8.

59. Yamka RM, Friesen KG, Frantz NZ. Identification of canine markers related to obesity and the effects of weight loss on the markers of interest. Intern J Appl Res Vet Med 2006;4:282–92.

60. Pena C, Suarez L, Bautista I, et al. Relationship between analytic values and canine obesity. J Anim Physiol Anim Nutr (Berl) 2008;92:324–5.

61. Yin N, Wang D, Zhang H, et al. Molecular mechanisms involved in the growth stimulation of breast cancer cells by leptin. Cancer Res 2004;64:5870–5.

62. Wang XJ, Yaun SL, Lu Q, et al. Potential involvement of leptin in carcinogenesis of hepatocellular carcinoma. World J Gastroenterol 2004;10:2478–81.

63. Glickman LT, Schofer FS, McKee LJ, et al. Epidemiologic study of insecticide exposures, obesity, and risk of bladder cancer in household dogs. J Toxicol Environ Health 1989;28:407–14.

64. Sonnenschein EG, Glickman LT, Goldschmidt MH, et al. Body conformation, diet, and risk of breast cancer in pet dogs: a case-controlled study. Am J Epidemiol 1991;133:694–703.

65. Perez Alenza D, Rutteman GR, Pena L, et al. Relation between habitual diet and canine mammary tumors in a case-control study. J Vet Intern Med 1998;12:132–9.

66. Philibert JC, Snyder PW, Glickman N, et al. Influence of host factors on survival in dogs with malignant mammary gland tumors. J Vet Intern Med 2003;17:102–6.

67. Lim HY, Im KS, Kim NH, et al. Effects of obesity and obesity-related molecules on canine mammary gland tumors. Vet Pathol 2015;52:1045–51.

68. Lim HY, Im KS, Kim NH, et al. Obesity, expression of adipocytokines, and macrophage infiltration in canine mammary tumors. Vet J 2015;203:326–31.

69. Weeth LP, Fascetti AJ, Kass PH, et al. Prevalence of obese dogs in a population of dogs with cancer. Am J Vet Res 2007;68:389–98.

70. Lawler DF, Evans RH, Larson BT, et al. Influence of lifetime food restriction on causes, time, and predictors of death in dogs. J Am Vet Med Assoc 2005;226:225–31.

71. Michel KE, Sorenmo K, Shofer FS. Evaluation of body condition and weight loss in dogs presented to a veterinary oncology service. J Vet Intern Med 2004;18:692–5.

72. Zhang X, Lerman LO. Obesity and renovascular disease. Am J Physiol Renal Physiol 2015;309:F273–9.

73. Chang Y, Ryu S, Choi Y, et al. Metabolically healthy obesity and development of chronic kidney disease: a cohort study. Ann Intern Med 2016;164(5):305–12.

74. Hunley TE, Ma LJ, Kon V. Scope and mechanisms of obesity-related renal disease. Curr Opin Nephrol Hypertens 2010;19:227–34.

75. Tirosh A, Golan R, Harman-Boehm I, et al. Renal function following three distinct weight loss dietary strategies during 2 years of a randomized controlled trial. Diabetes Care 2013;36:2225–32.

76. Jesudason DR, Pedersen E, Clifton PM. Weight-loss diets in people with type 2 diabetes and renal disease: a randomized controlled trial of the effect of different dietary protein amounts. Am J Clin Nutr 2013;98:494–501.

77. Lohmeier TE, Iliescu R, Liu B, et al. Systemic and renal-specific sympathoinhibition in obesity hypertension. Hypertension 2012;59:331–8.

78. Heneger JR, Bigler SA, Heneger LK, et al. Functional and structural changes in the kidney in the early stages of obesity. J Am Soc Nephrol 2001;12:1211–7.

79. Tvarijonaviciute A, Ceron JJ, Holden SL, et al. Effect of weight loss in obese dogs on indicators of renal function or disease. J Vet Intern Med 2013;27:31–8.

80. Tefft KM, Shaw DH, Ihle SL, et al. Association between excess body weight and urine protein concentration in healthy dogs. Vet Clin Pathol 2014;43:255–66.

81. D'Elia JA, Roshan B, Maski M, et al. Manifestation of renal disease in obesity: pathophysiology of obesity-related dysfunction of the kidney. Int J Nephrol Renovas Dis 2009;2:39–49.

82. Warren BS, Wakshlag JJ, Miley M, et al. Use of pedometers to measure the relationship of dog walking to body condition score in obese and non-obese dogs. Br J Nutr 2011;106:S85–9.

83. Morrison R, Penprave V, Beber A, et al. Associations between obesity and physical activity in dogs: a preliminary investigation. J Small Anim Pract 2013;54:570–4.

84. Fontaine KR, Barofsky I, Anderson RE, et al. Impact of weight loss on health-related quality of life. Qual Life Res 1999;8:275–7.

85. Fine JT, Colditz GA, Coakley EH, et al. A prospective study of weight change and health-related quality of life in women. J Am Med Assoc 1999;282:2136–42.

86. German AJ, Holden SL, Wiseman-Orr ML, et al. Quality of life is reduced in obese dogs but improves after successful weight loss. Vet J 2012;192:428–34.

87. Wiseman-Orr ML, Nolan AM, Reid J, et al. Development of a questionnaire to measure the effects of chronic pain on health-related quality of life in dogs. Am J Vet Res 2004;65:1077–84.
88. Mlacnik E, Bockstahler BA, Muller M, et al. Effects of caloric restriction and moderate or intense physiotherapy program for treatment of lameness in overweight dogs with osteoarthritis. J Am Vet Med Assoc 2006;229:1756–60.
89. Marshall WG, Hazewinkel HA, Mullen D, et al. The effect of weight loss on lameness in obese dogs with osteoarthritis. Vet Res Commun 2010;34:241–53.
90. Weindruch R. The retardation of aging by calorie restriction: studies in rodents and primates. Toxicol Pathol 1996;24:742–5.
91. Fonarow GC, Srikanthan P, Costanzo MR, et al. An obesity paradox in acute heart failure: analysis of body mass index and inhospital mortality for 108927 patients in the Acute Decompensated Heart Failure National Registry. Am Heart J 2007;153: 74–81.
92. Webster G, Zhang J, Rosenthal R. Comparison of the epidemiology and co-morbidities of heart failure in the pediatric and adult populations: a retrospective, cross-sectional study. BMC Cardiovasc Disord 2006;6:23–9.
93. Curtis JP, Setler JG, Wang Y, et al. The obesity paradox: body mass index and outcomes in patients with heart failure. Arch Intern Med 2005;165:55–61.
94. Finn E, Freeman LM, Rush JE, et al. The relationship between body weight, body condition, and survival in cats with heart failure. J Vet Intern Med 2010;24: 1369–74.
95. Slupe JL, Freeman LM, Rush JE. Association of body weight and body condition with survival in dogs with heart failure. J Vet Intern Med 2008;22:561–5.
96. Parker VJ, Freeman LM. Association between body condition and survival in dogs with acquired chronic kidney disease. J Vet Intern Med 2011;25:1306–11.
97. Webster J, Hesp R, Garrow J. The composition of excess weight in obese women estimated by body density, total body water and total body potassium. Hum Nutr Clin Nutr 1984;38:299–306.

Nutritional Assessment

Laura Eirmann, DVM[a],[b],*

KEYWORDS

- Canine • Feline • Obesity • Nutritional assessment • Diet history

KEY POINTS

- Nutritional assessment is an iterative process that includes animal-specific factors, diet-specific factors, feeding management, and environmental factors.
- The nutritional assessment is an essential component of every patient visit during each veterinary consultation.
- The nutritional assessment includes a medical history, thorough diet history, and complete physical examination with appropriate diagnostic testing.
- A comprehensive nutritional assessment lays the foundation for developing a successful treatment plan for the overweight or obese patient.

INTRODUCTION

Nutritional assessment is an iterative process that encompasses evaluation of the animal, the food being offered and consumed, the animal's environment, and the feeding management strategy being used by the caregiver. These factors are interrelated and are depicted by the American College of Veterinary Nutrition "Circle of Nutrition" (**Fig. 1**). The American Hospital Association and the World Small Animal Veterinary Association recommend nutritional assessment and dietary recommendations every time a pet presents for veterinary consultation.[1,2] Each factor influences the patient's nutritional status and because each factor can change over time, reassessment of each variable and possible modification of the nutrition plan is warranted. When presented with an overweight or obese pet, the nutrition assessment is an essential starting point. Careful consideration of animal-specific, diet-specific, feeding management, and environmental factors allows the clinician to develop a specific nutrition plan for that patient that is acceptable and achievable to the owner and the pet.

PATIENT ASSESSMENT

Relevant animal-specific factors are obtained during patient assessment. Signalment is important because certain endogenous patient variables can increase the risk of an

Disclosures: The author has nothing to disclose.
[a] Nutrition Service, Oradell Animal Hospital, 580 Winters Avenue, Paramus, NJ 07652, USA;
[b] Veterinary Communications, Nestlé Purina PetCare, Checkerboard Square, St Louis, MO 63164, USA
* Oradell Animal Hospital, 580 Winters Avenue, Paramus, NJ 07652.
E-mail address: leirmann@oradell.com

Vet Clin Small Anim 46 (2016) 855–867
http://dx.doi.org/10.1016/j.cvsm.2016.04.012
0195-5616/16/$ – see front matter © 2016 Elsevier Inc. All rights reserved.

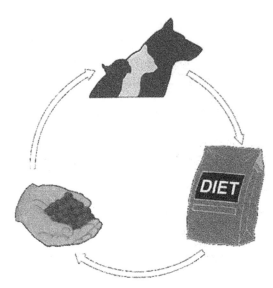

Fig. 1. The animal, diet, and feeding management are each evaluated during a nutritional assessment. These factors are interrelated. (*Courtesy of* the American College of Veterinary Nutrition, Santa Clarita, CA; with permission.)

animal becoming obese. Certain breeds of dogs (eg, Labrador Retriever, Cocker Spaniel, Dachshund, Shetland Sheepdog, Golden Retriever)[3] and cats (eg, Domestic Shorthair, Manx)[4] may be predisposed to becoming overweight or obese, although specific genetic factors leading to obesity are complex and are not currently completely understood. Middle-aged dogs and cats are at an increased risk for being overweight.[3,4] Neutering can alter energy balance and increase food intake resulting in weight gain.[5–14] Although the patient's signalment cannot be changed, recognition of endogenous risk factors that may predispose to obesity should be discussed at an early stage with the pet owner so that appropriate modifications to the nutrition plan, such as decreasing energy intake at the time of neutering, can be instituted.

Medical History

A complete medical history is an important component of the nutritional assessment. The patient may be suffering from one of several comorbidities associated with obesity that may impact diet selection (eg, lower carbohydrate intake for a diabetic cat) or impact the overall weight loss plan (eg, concurrent physical therapy for an arthritic dog). Certain endocrinopathies, such as hypothyroidism or hyperadrenocorticism, can contribute to weight gain. Some medications can contribute to weight gain either by causing polyphagia (eg, phenobarbital) or by altering protein, carbohydrate, and lipid metabolism resulting in weight gain and increased adiposity (eg, glucocorticoids). An essential component of the comprehensive history is a thorough dietary history, discussed in more detail in a later section.

Physical Examination

A comprehensive physical examination is an integral component of the nutritional assessment. Comorbidities that limit exercise tolerance or necessitate specific nutrient modification impact the nutrition plan. The pet's body weight must be documented in the medical record during every patient visit.

Body condition assessment

Although body weight and body weight trends over time provide an objective measurement, body weight alone does not provide any indication of adiposity or body composition, such as lean/fat mass ratio. Because obesity can be defined as an excess of body fat sufficient to result in impaired health,[15] the veterinarian must evaluate the animal's degree of adiposity (the fat mass component of the patient's body composition). There are various methods for evaluating body composition including dual-energy x-ray absorptiometry, bioelectric impedance analysis, and total body water determined by deuterium oxide dilution technique that are used in research settings. However in the clinical examination room, the practical, inexpensive, noninvasive morphometric methods, such as body condition scoring, are recommended. Body condition scoring relies on visual assessment and palpation of specific body regions including the rib cage, waist and lumbar region, and base of the tail. This assessment provides a semiquantitative method of evaluating body composition. Several scoring systems have been developed and evaluated in dogs and cats.[16–20] The veterinary hospital should train all staff to use one agreed on system and consistently assess and record body condition score for each patient during each examination. **Figs. 2** and **3** depict a nine-point system that has been validated for repeatability and reproducibility between trained observers.[16,17,21,22] Using this system, each unit increase in body condition score above ideal is approximately equivalent to 10% to 15% over ideal body weight.[23] In addition to the clinical use of body condition scoring, this technique can be taught to pet owners allowing them to evaluate their pet at home. The World Small Animal Association's Global Nutrition Committee Web site provides a link to a body condition score video (https://www.youtube.com/watch?v=tf_-rwxqHYU&feature=youtu.be).

Muscle condition assessment

Body condition scoring assesses fat mass. It does not provide an indication of muscle or lean body mass. Muscle condition scoring evaluates muscle mass and is independent of body condition score. An obese animal may have evidence of muscle loss. A muscle scoring system has been developed for dogs and cats and to date has been evaluated in cats.[24] **Fig. 4** depicts a muscle scoring system based on palpation of the skeletal musculature over the spine, skull, scapula, and pelvis. Loss of muscle mass may indicate an underlying disease condition that should be investigated before finalizing a nutrition plan. Evaluating muscle mass as part of the initial nutritional assessment and reassessing as the obese patient loses weight is recommended because the goal is to maintain lean body mass while the patient loses excessive body fat.

General Diagnostic Testing

Routine laboratory evaluation including a complete blood count, serum biochemistry, and urinalysis is recommended to further evaluate the health status of the patient. Additional diagnostic testing based on historical and physical examination findings may be indicated before a nutrition plan is developed. For instance, historical or physical examination findings may prompt further testing for conditions, such as hypothyroidism or hyperadrenocorticism, which may have predisposed to weight gain.

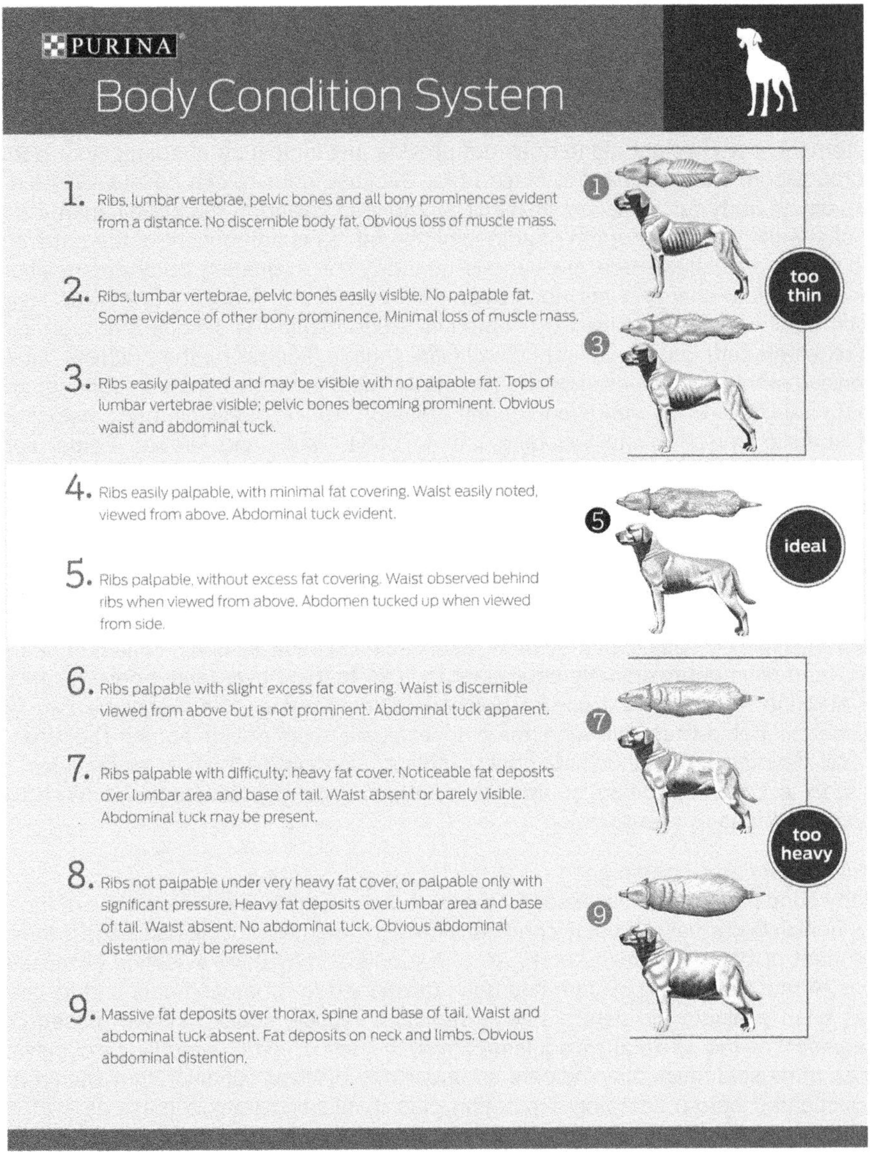

Fig. 2. Nine-point body condition scoring system for dogs. (*Courtesy of* Nestle Purina Pet-Care Company, St Louis, MO; with permission.)

DIET ASSESSMENT
Obtain a Complete Diet History

A comprehensive diet history is a critical component of the nutritional assessment of an overweight or obese patient. The detailed information that should be obtained during a diet history is outlined in **Box 1**. To facilitate obtaining a comprehensive diet history, a form can be provided to the owner before the appointment. This allows the caregivers an opportunity to look at pet food labels at home, measure the amount

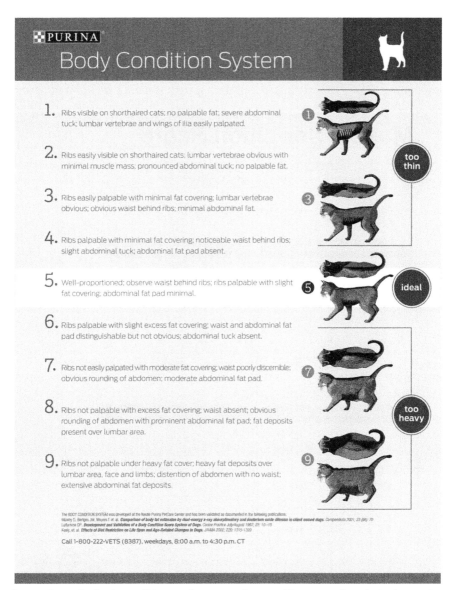

Fig. 3. Nine-point body condition scoring system for cats. (*Courtesy of* Nestle Purina PetCare Company, St Louis, MO; with permission.)

they are feeding, and perhaps keep a food diary before the consultation. The author's veterinary hospital provides on-line access to a diet history form (**Fig. 5**) and requests owners complete and return the form before the nutrition consultation. This allows the veterinary team to review the information, prepare clarifying questions, and obtain calorie information before the visit. The diet history form should complement but not replace the owner interview. The owner interview is an essential component of the nutritional assessment and is discussed in more detail later in this article.

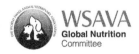

Muscle Condition Score

Muscle condition score is assessed by visualization and palpation of the spine, scapulae, skull, and wings of the ilia. Muscle loss is typically first noted in the epaxial muscles on each side of the spine; muscle loss at other sites can be more variable. Muscle condition score is graded as normal, mild loss, moderate loss, or severe loss. Note that animals can have significant muscle loss even if they are overweight (body condition score >5/9). Conversely, animals can have a low body condition score (<4/9) but have minimal muscle loss. Therefore, assessing both body condition score and muscle condition score on every animal at every visit is important. Palpation is especially important with mild muscle loss and in animals that are overweight. An example of each score is shown below.

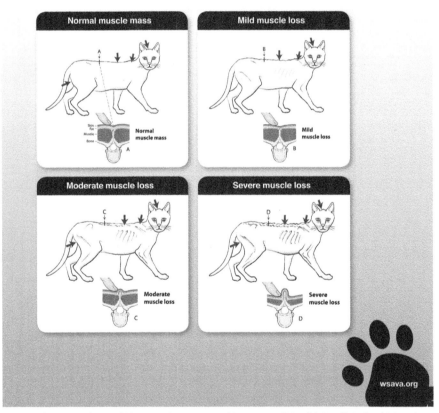

Fig. 4. Feline muscle condition scoring system. (*Courtesy of* World Small Animal Veterinary Association, Ontario, Canada; with permission.)

Estimate Current Energy Intake

Depending on the level of detail provided in the diet history, the pet's current calorie intake can be estimated. Calorie information for commercial pet food and treats is available via the product label, manufacturer's product guide, Web site, or the customer service department. Calorie content of human foods is found on the

---

Box 1
Diet history outline

- What does the pet currently eat?
  - Exact brand and variety (flavor) of all commercial pet foods
  - Recipes if a home-prepared meal is fed
  - Specific table foods or scraps
  - Commercial dog treats and all other between meal snacks (biscuits, rawhides, foods used to fill interactive feeding toys, and so forth)
  - Chew toys, such as bully sticks and bones
  - Treats or products provided for dental health
  - Dietary supplements
  - All flavored medications and foods used to give medication
  - Other food sources (outdoor hunting, scavenging, access to neighbor's pet food)
  - "Special occasion foods" (a weekly treat, special meal after a trip to the veterinarian, and so forth)

- How is food offered and how much does the pet consume?
  - Free choice or meal fed
  - If meal fed:
    - Number of meals per day
    - Portion of meal when known; if a volumetric measuring device is used document the size of the "scoop" or "cup" or the size of the can
  - Document the quantity of every food item the pet consumes (the size of a commercial treat and the number fed per day, the amount of food used hide a medication, and so forth)

- When and where does the pet eat?
  - Timing and location of meals (fed from the table, a food bowl, a food puzzle, and so forth)
  - Timing of between meal foods and purpose (training treats, interactive feeding toy provided when owner leaves the home, and so forth)
  - Other pets present during feeding (competitive feeding behaviors or access to other pets' food)
  - Foods given during the owner's food preparation or family meal time (feeding from dinner table)
  - Unsupervised access to food (outdoor scavenging, hunting, and so forth)

- Who feeds the pet?
  - Number of people and other animals in the household
    - Primary or multiple individuals who provide meals or snacks
    - Individuals who may provide unintended food (eg, child dropping food from the highchair, access to the cat's food)
  - Individuals not living in the household who may provide food (dog walker, trainer, groomer, friends at the dog park, and so forth)

Nutrition Facts label on the packaging or by looking up caloric information on Web sites, such as the US Department of Agriculture's National Nutrient Database (http://ndb.nal.usda.gov/ndb/search). An estimated daily caloric intake provides valuable information. The veterinarian can determine if the reported daily energy intake seems exceedingly low. This may indicate inaccurate measurement, unaccounted access to additional food, or a patient with a rather low metabolic rate. There is considerable variation in daily energy requirements among individuals.[25,26] Knowing a specific pet's daily energy requirement based on an accurate diet history can help determine an initial daily calorie recommendation for weight loss for that individual.

Evaluate Current Nutrient Intake

The diet history can determine if the pet's nutrient needs are being met. Aside from ensuring the food is complete and balanced for the animal's life stage, one can

Pet's Name:

Breed: Age:

Owner's Name:

Diet History Form
DATE:_____
Current body weight:_____Usual body weight:_____
Do you consider your pet: Overweight ____Underweight ____ Ideal____
Reason for Nutrition Consultation
_____

Please list all food(s) you currently feed at mealtime. Include ALL commercial pet foods. If you add human food items to a commercial food, please list that as well. If you cook for your pet provide the detailed recipe (for example "4 ounces of 85% lean ground beef pan-fried & 1 cup of cooked long-grain brown rice daily") *The description should provide enough detail that the reader could purchase the same food or prepare the exact recipe.*

Meals: Brand/Product/Food	Amount Fed Form	Per Meal	# of Meals	Flavor	Fed Since
EXAMPLES:					
Purina Dog Chow Healthy Morsels	dry	1 1/2 cups	twice a day	chicken and rice	May 2013
Boneless Chicken (white meat)	boiled	2 ounces	three times a week		June 2015

List all treats & "between meal snacks" include biscuits, pet treats, rawhides, pig's ears, table foods etc. Anything given as a "snack" or "treat"

Brand/Product/Treat	Size	Flavor	Quantity Per Day	Fed Since
EXAMPLES:				
Greenies	small	regular	twice per week	April 2012
Milk Bones	medium	beef	three per day	June 2013
Kraft Non-fat American Cheese	slice	--	two per day	May 2015

Please describe pet's activity level (i.e. type, duration & frequency): _____
Do you have other pets? ☐ Yes ☐ No   If so, please list (species, age): _____
Do you have children in the home? ☐ Yes ☐ No
Is your pet fed in the presence of other animals? ☐ Yes ☐ No
If yes, please describe: _____
Does your pet have access to other unmonitored food sources (i.e. food from a neighbor, scavenging from the yard/trash, hunting outdoors, etc.)? ☐ Yes ☐ No If yes, please describe: _____
Who typically feeds your pet? _____
How do you store your pet's food? _____
Do you use food to administer medication? If yes please describe type of food and amount: _____
Please describe anything you give your pet for dental health (treats, dental chews, bones or similar products): _____

If you brush your pet's teeth, please list the toothpaste you use (if any): _____

Please list other foods your pet has received in the past but is NOT currently eating, indicating the approximate time period when they were fed. *Examples are given in italics.*

Brand/Product/Food	Form	From	To	Reason Stopped
EXAMPLE:				
Hill's Science Diet Feline Growth	can	June 2006	March 2007	became an adult

Please list the name of each additional nutritional supplement your pet receives, indicate how much and how often your pet receives it (i.e. herbal product, fatty acid, vitamin or mineral supplement): _____

Please list your pet's current and past medical problems, date/year diagnosed, and whether the condition has resolved or not: _____

Please list all medications your pet is currently receiving (indicate doses/strengths and frequency): _____

Please check the box, and indicate frequency, if the following problems have been experienced by your pet prior to today's visit:
   ☐ Recent involuntary or unintended ☐ weight gain **OR** ☐ weight loss
   ☐ How many pounds? _____ Over what time period: _____
☐ Vomiting   _____ times/day   _____ times/week
☐ Diarrhea   _____ times/day   _____ times/week

Have you observed changes in any of the following:
☐ Urination **OR** ☐ Drinking   What was the specific change? _____Since when? _____
☐ Defecation   What was the specific change? _____Since when? _____
☐ Appetite   What was the specific change? _____Since when? _____

Does your pet have? ☐ allergies **OR** difficulty ☐ chewing ☐ swallowing
If so, please describe:_____

Fig. 5. Sample diet history form.

determine if the food is being fed in an appropriate amount to meet nutrient needs. Sometimes owners perceive even an overweight pet as "picky" so a significant amount of table food is added to a complete and balanced commercial pet food to entice the pet to eat. Aside from adding additional calories, these food sources typically do not provide all essential nutrients. Consuming table foods and snacks in excess of 10% of the total daily energy intake may result in an overall unbalanced diet.[1] The caregiver may be providing dental chews, supplements, or foods to hide medications that contribute a significant amount of calories without considering the impact of these items on the pet's daily caloric intake. Variables, such as the number of snacks, feeding table scraps, and the dog's presence when the owners prepare or eat their own meals, have been associated with canine obesity.[27–29] Although most animal-specific endogenous risk factors associated with obesity cannot be modified, a thorough diet history can reveal certain exogenous risk factors related to the food and feeding management that can be modified.

Owner Interview

Although a diet history form can provide important information, it complements but does not replace the owner interview. A conversation with the pet's caretaker expands on the information obtained on the diet history form and provides more insight on the family's perspective of the pet's nutritional and health status. The type of questioning can influence the information provided by the pet owner. A recent qualitative conversation analytical study concluded that "what-prefaced" questions focusing on the main commercial food (ie, "What do you feed your pet?") is the predominant format used to initiate the diet history.[30] The researchers noted this format resulted in a brief "checklist" dialogue that could negatively impact the accuracy and completeness of the nutritional history. Therefore they recommend initially engaging the owner in a narrative by asking broader "telling" questions, such as "Tell me about your pet's typical day," followed by increasingly more specific questions including "Tell me about your pet's normal eating habits."[30] Communication skills that involve asking questions, rephrasing responses, and clarifying information in an empathetic manner involve the owner and help the veterinarian not only elicit details about the pet and the home environment but also provide a framework for communicating the nutritional recommendation.

Current Feeding Management and Environment

Although food-specific details, such as the brand of pet food, are a necessary component of the nutritional assessment, equally important is an understanding of the feeding management (husbandry) and the pet's environment. The diet history includes not only what the pet eats and how much, but also includes details regarding who feeds the pet, how the pet is fed, and where and when the pet is fed. The environment includes access to the outdoors and opportunity to exercise. If the pet goes outdoors unsupervised, the possibility of access to unmonitored food sources must be considered. Environmental factors associated with obesity include less exercise or play,[28,29,31] confinement to a yard rather than leash walking,[28] and indoor confinement for cats.[32]

The Role Food Plays in the Pet-Owner Relationship

The owner interview provides an opportunity to learn more about the role food plays in pet and family member interactions. For example, a special weekly food treat may be an important interaction with this pet. The veterinarian or technician should ask who lives in the household and whether one or multiple individuals provide the meals and snacks. If multiple individuals feed the pet or if one individual has a special feeding ritual with the pet, certain strategies may need to be discussed when the nutrition plan is developed.

Rather than asking, "Do you feed treats?" open-ended questions, such as "Tell me about the snacks your pet enjoys" and "Describe how you reward your pet when he is at obedience class" often provide more detail about specific food items and more insight into the role food plays in the pet-owner interactions. Inquiring about the pet's daily routine can reveal specific food-pet-owner interactions, such as a bedtime snack or a daily treat when the mail is delivered. Learning more about the routine during mealtime may provide insight about the owner's concerns over the pet's eating behaviors. For instance, owners who watch their pet eat are more likely to have an obese dog or cat.[27,31] It is not uncommon for a concerned owner of an overweight dog who watches the pet very closely at mealtime to express concern that the pet does not like a certain food or is a picky eater.

Owner's Interest and Willingness to Change to Help the Pet Lose Weight

An accurate assessment of the pet's body condition score by the veterinarian is not sufficient if the owner does not recognize the pet is overweight or obese. Multiple studies have concluded that owners of overweight pets do not perceive the pet is overweight and underestimate their pet's body condition.[29,33–37] A critical component of nutritional assessment involves assessment of the caregiver. Does this owner perceive the pet as overweight? Does the owner understand why weight loss is recommended? Is the owner still contemplating weight loss or are they ready to proceed with dietary changes and a change in the feeding routine?

Identify Potential Opportunities and Challenges for Successful Weight Loss

During the nutritional assessment the veterinarian should identify and consider opportunities and challenges the pet and family may face at home before proceeding to a detailed nutrition recommendation and treatment plan. Discovering what motivates a client can provide the perfect opportunity to discuss weight loss and the health benefits for that pet. The owner seeking ways to improve an obese arthritic pet's mobility may be motivated by learning that weight loss can often improve mobility.[38–40] Conversely there may be issues that will make weight loss more difficult. A family member may not agree that the pet is overweight or does not appreciate the health risks associated with obesity. The owner may have tried a weight loss plan in the past that did not work. Recognizing these challenges allows the clinician to tailor a plan to meet the needs of the pet and the family.[41]

SUMMARY

Nutritional assessment is a necessary component of every veterinary consultation. For the obese patient it is an essential tool to obtain specific information about the pet, the foods the pet consumes, the caregivers, and the pet's environment. The process involves a detailed history that requires strong client communication skills and excellent medical and technical skills to perform a complete medical examination with appropriate diagnostic testing. A comprehensive nutritional assessment provides the foundation for developing a successful treatment plan for the overweight or obese patient.

REFERENCES

1. Baldwin K, Bartges J, Buffington T, et al. AAHA nutritional assessment guidelines for dogs and cats. J Am Anim Hosp Assoc 2010;46:285–96.
2. Freeman L, Becvarova I, Cave N, et al. WSAVA nutritional assessment guidelines. J Small Anim Pract 2011;52:385–96.
3. Lund EM, Armstrong PJ, Kirk CA, et al. Prevalence and risk factors for obesity in adult dogs from private US veterinary practices. Intern J Appl Res Vet Med 2006; 4:177–86.
4. Lund EM, Armstrong PJ, Kirk CA, et al. Prevalence and risk factors for obesity in adult cats from private US veterinary practices. Int J Appl Res Vet Med 2005;3: 88–95.
5. Houpt KA, Coren B, Hintz HF, et al. Effect of sex and reproductive status on sucrose preference, food intake, and body weight of dogs. J Am Vet Med Assoc 1979;174:1083–5.
6. Root M, Johnson S, Olson P. Effect of prepuberal and postpuberal gonadectomy and heat production measured by indirect calorimetry in male and female domestic cats. Am J Vet Res 1996;57:1–4.
7. Fettman M, Stanton C, Banks L, et al. Effects of neutering on bodyweight, metabolic rate and glucose tolerance of domestic cats. Res Vet Sci 1997; 62:131–6.
8. Jeusette I, Detilleux J, Cuvelier C, et al. Ad libitum feeding following ovariectomy in female Beagle dogs: effect on maintenance energy requirement and on blood metabolites. J Anim Physiol Anim Nutr (Berl) 2004;88:117–21.
9. Jeusette I, Daminet S, Nguyen P, et al. Effect of ovariectomy and ad libitum feeding on body composition, thyroid status, ghrelin and leptin plasma concentrations in female dogs. J Anim Physiol Anim Nutr (Berl) 2006;90:12–8.
10. Flynn MF, Hardie EM, Armstrong PJ. Effect of ovariohysterectomy on maintenance energy requirement in cats. J Am Vet Med Assoc 1996;209: 1572–81.
11. Harper EJ, Stack DM, Watson TD, et al. Effects of feeding regimens on bodyweight, composition and condition score in cats following ovariohysterectomy. J Small Anim Pract 2001;42:433–8.
12. Belsito K, Vester B, Keel T, et al. Impact of ovariohysterectomy and food intake on body composition, physical activity, and adipose gene expression in cats. J Anim Sci 2009;87:594–602.
13. Kanchuk M, Backus R, Calvert C, et al. Weight gain in gonadectomized normal and lipoprotein lipase-deficient male domestic cats results from increased food intake and not decreased energy expenditure. J Nutr 2003;133:1866–74.
14. Lefebvre SL, Yang M, Wang M, et al. Effect of age at gonadectomy on the probability of dogs becoming overweight. J Am Vet Med Assoc 2013;243: 236–43.
15. Laflamme D. Understanding and managing obesity in dogs and cats. Vet Clin North Am 2006;36:1283–95.
16. Laflamme D. Development and validation of a body condition score system for dogs. Canine Pract 1997;22:10–5.
17. Laflamme D. Development and validation of a body condition score system for cats: a clinical tool. Feline Pract 1997;25:13–8.
18. German A, Holden S, Moxham G, et al. A simple, reliable tool for owners to assess the body condition of their dog or cat. J Nutr 2006;136:2031S–3S.

19. Witzel A, Kirk C, Henry G, et al. Use of a morphometric method and body fat index system for estimation of body composition in overweight and obese dogs. J Am Vet Med Assoc 2014;244:1279–84.
20. Witzel A, Kirk C, Henry G, et al. Use of a morphometric method and body fat index system for estimation of body composition in overweight and obese cats. J Am Vet Med Assoc 2014;224:1285–90.
21. Mawby D, Bartges J, d'Avignon A, et al. Comparison of various methods for estimating body fat in dogs. J Am Anim Hosp Assoc 2004;40:109–14.
22. Bjornvad C, Nielsen D, Armstrong P, et al. Evaluation of a nine-point body condition scoring system in physically inactive pet cats. Am J Vet Res 2011;72:433–7.
23. Laflamme D. Companion Animals Symposium: obesity in dogs and cats: What is wrong with being fat? J Anim Sci 2012;90:1653–62.
24. Michel K, Anderson W, Cupp C, et al. Correlation of a feline muscle mass score with body composition determined by dual-energy X-ray absoptiometry. Br J Nutr 2011;106:57S–9S.
25. Laflamme D, Kuhlman G, Lawler D. Evaluation of weight loss protocols for dogs. J Am Anim Hosp Assoc 1997;33:253–9.
26. Butterwick R, Hawthorne A. Advances in dietary management of obesity in dogs and cats. J Nutr 1998;128:2771S–5S.
27. Kienzle E, Bergler R, Mandernach A. A comparison of the feeding behavior and the human-animal relationship in owners of normal and obese dogs. J Nutr 1998;128:2779S–82S.
28. Bland I, Guthrie-Jones A, Taylor R, et al. Dog obesity: owner attitudes and behaviour. Prev Vet Med 2009;92:333–40.
29. Courcier E, Thomson R, Mellor D, et al. An epidemiological study of environmental factors associated with canine obesity. J Small Anim Pract 2010;51:362–7.
30. MacMartin C, Wheat H, Coe J, et al. Effect of question design on dietary information solicited during veterinarian-client interactions in companion animal practice in Ontario, Canada. J Am Vet Med Assoc 2015;246:1203–13.
31. Kienzle E, Bergler R. Human-animal relationship of owners of normal and overweight cats. J Nutr 2006;136:1947S–50S.
32. Rowe E, Browne W, Casey R, et al. Risk factors identified for owner-reported feline obesity at around one year of age: dry diet and indoor lifestyle. Prev Vet Med 2015;121:273–81.
33. Singh R, Laflamme D, Sidebottom-Nielsen M. Owner perception of canine body condition score. J Vet Intern Med 2002;16:362.
34. White GA, Hobson-West P, Cobb K, et al. Canine obesity: is there a difference between veterinarian and owner perception? J Small Anim Pract 2011;52:622–6.
35. Rohlf V, Toukhsati S, Coleman G, et al. Dog obesity: can dog caregivers' (owners') feeding and exercise intentions and behaviors be predicted from attitudes? J Appl Anim Welf Sci 2010;13:213–36.
36. Colliard L, Paragon B, Lemuet B, et al. Prevalence and risk factors of obesity in an urban population of healthy cats. J Feline Med Surg 2009;11:135–40.
37. Cave N, Allan F, Schokkenbroek S, et al. A cross-sectional study to compare changes in the prevalence and risk factors for feline obesity between 1993 and 2007 in New Zealand. Prev Vet Med 2012;107:121–33.
38. Impellizeri J, Tetrick M, Muir P. Effect of weight reduction on clinical signs of lameness in dogs with hip osteoarthritis. J Am Vet Med Assoc 2000;216:1089–91.

39. Marshall W, Hazewinkel H, Mullen D, et al. The effect of weight loss on lameness in obese dogs with osteoarthritis. Vet Res Commun 2010;34:241–53.
40. Mlacnik E, Bockstahler B, Muller M, et al. Effects of caloric restriction and a moderate or intense physiotherapy program for treatment of lameness in overweight dogs with osteoarthritis. J Am Vet Med Assoc 2006;229:1756–60.
41. Brooks D, Churchill J, Fein K, et al. 2014 AAHA weight management guidelines for dogs and cats. J Am Anim Hosp Assoc 2014;50:1–11.

Dietary Aspects of Weight Management in Cats and Dogs

Deborah E. Linder, DVM[a],*, Valerie J. Parker, DVM[b]

KEYWORDS

- Obesity • Nutrition • Client communication • Macronutrients • Micronutrients
- Optimal nutrient profile

KEY POINTS

- The optimal weight loss diet is best informed by obtaining a full dietary history and performing a detailed assessment of the pet, pet owner, and environment in which the pet lives.
- Dietary selection is guided by macronutrient and micronutrient needs of each cat or dog.
- Adjusting the rate of weight loss and calorie restriction requires frequent follow-up, and owners should be prepared for multiple weigh-ins to adequately align expectations and timeframe for weight loss.
- An important component of successful weight management is the role that human–pet relationships can play in affecting obesity treatment and adherence to dietary management.
- Because weight management plans can be labor intensive, veterinarians can use premade resources, such as frequently asked question handouts on nutrition-related myths or owner-directed guides for selecting pet foods.

INTRODUCTION

Choice of an optimal weight loss diet for cats and dogs is informed by obtaining a diet history and performing a detailed assessment of the pet, pet owner, and environment in which the pet lives. Incorporating information about pet and pet owner preferences can allow for individualization of the weight management plan and has the potential to increase adherence. There is no single best diet for every overweight pet, but there are several factors, medical and nonmedical, that should be considered before making a

Disclosure Statement: Dr D.E. Linder has received research funding within the past year from Zoetis, and has received consulting funding within the past year from Nestle Purina PetCare, Mars, and Banfield. Dr V.J. Parker has nothing to disclose.

[a] Department of Clinical Sciences, Cummings School of Veterinary Medicine at Tufts University, 200 Westboro Road, North Grafton, MA 01536, USA; [b] Department of Veterinary Clinical Sciences, The Ohio State University, 601 Vernon L. Tharp Street, Columbus, OH 43210, USA
* Corresponding author.
E-mail address: Deborah.Linder@tufts.edu

http://dx.doi.org/10.1016/j.cvsm.2016.04.008
0195-5616/16/$ – see front matter © 2016 Elsevier Inc. All rights reserved.
vetsmall.theclinics.com

diet recommendation as part of a weight management plan that will be discussed. Macronutrient considerations, including protein, fat, and carbohydrate content as well as nutrient and calorie density should be incorporated. An important component of successful weight management is the role that human–pet relationships can play in affecting obesity treatment and adherence to the diet plan decided on by the veterinarian and owner together. This article guides the veterinary health care team to work with the client to develop an individualized and optimal diet management plan for healthy cats and dogs, with recommendations for when to seek additional help from a board-certified veterinary nutritionist.

INITIAL APPROACH TO SELECTING THE OPTIMAL DIET

A complete nutritional assessment (see Laura Eirmann's article, "Nutritional Assessment," in this issue) is the basis for choosing the most appropriate weight loss diet for cats and dogs. Incorporating information about pet and pet owner preferences can allow for individualization of the weight management plan and has the potential to increase adherence.

Pet Assessment

Every pet should undergo physical examination and nutritional assessment (see Laura Eirmann's article, "Nutritional Assessment," in this issue). Clinicopathologic data and medical diagnostic workup as indicated is useful to elucidate comorbidities that may influence diet selection. Body condition score and muscle condition score are crucial parts of every examination and may also impact diet selection.[1–3] For example, a pet with severe muscle wasting has more specific protein needs, and one with a body condition score of 9 (9-point scale) may require severe, long-term calorie restriction, which warrants attention to nutrient density. Veterinarians should note that body condition score and muscle condition score may be discordant (ie, an obese pet could have severe muscle wasting).

Impact of Diet History

A complete diet history allows for an accurate estimate of calorie intake. For examples of published diet history forms (see Laura Eirmann's article, "Nutritional Assessment," in this issue).[4,5] Many owners are unaware that supplements, treats, rawhides and dental chews provide calories, so these should be discussed. For example, more than half of pet owners administer medication in a food item[6] and often do not recognize this part of the pet's diet without further questioning. In the authors' experience, pet owners commonly use high-calorie food items such as margarine or peanut butter to assist in administering medication. All owners should be counseled on recommended food items and portion for medication administration.

Obtaining information through a complete diet history may inform diet selection because of preferences of the pet owner. For example, some diet options may have nutrients or additives that would otherwise be given as supplements (eg, glucosamine for osteoarthritis, which is a common comorbidity with obesity). Eliminating additional supplements may simplify management and improve client adherence. Further, knowing that a pet owner has concerns about the pet's dental health allows for discussion of tooth brushing or selection of diets formulated to improve dental health (ie, with Veterinary Oral Health Council seal of acceptance; www.vohc.org), while removing incentive for owners to give treats or chews with dental health claims that may add unnecessary calories or unbalance the diet. Most importantly, obtaining a diet history allows for an understanding of owner preferences and "non-negotiables," which may impact the diet plan. Non-negotiables are food items or parts of the pet–owner relationship that owners will continue to employ regardless of what veterinarians recommend or regardless of what they report to veterinarians. Diet history can elucidate what is most important to pet owners, allowing these aspects to be incorporated into the diet management plan to improve adherence.

Owner Assessment

After assessing the pet and obtaining a complete diet history, taking time to fully understand the environment and pet owners allows for assessment of the owner's readiness to change and ability to adhere to a diet plan. (See Julie Churchill and Ernie Ward's article, "Communicating with Pet Owners About Obesity: Roles of the Veterinary Health Care Team," in this issue.) Some pet owners may not be ready and are still contemplating weight management for their pet. In these situations, client education and monitoring may be the best course of action before engaging in a full weight loss program. However, those preparing or taking action for weight management in their pet would best benefit from specific individualized plans and feedback.[7] For example, pet owners may think that they just need to pick a diet food but are not sure which diet to select, what amount to feed, and how to address treats outside the main diet. Providing vague directions, such as "switch to a light food" or "cut back a little on the kibble," is not effective and can increase confusion for pet owners.[8] Engaging pet owners and understanding their readiness to change can impact the weight loss plan and diet selection. Guidance on assessing readiness to change has been described elsewhere (see Julie Churchill and Ernie Ward's article, "Communicating with Pet Owners About Obesity: Roles of the Veterinary Health Care Team," in this issue).[7] Although initiating the conversation with owners about their pets' weight can be challenging, understanding the pet owner's perspective can guide management, and talking tips have been described to assist the veterinary health care team in these discussions.[9]

Through these discussions, owners may relay that they would be interested in pursuing any plan that the veterinarian recommends, or they may explain their level or ability of commitment, which could guide weight management and diet selection. For owners that are interested in any type of plan, veterinarians can focus solely on medical factors that would guide management. However, in other instances, veterinarians may need to balance medical and nonmedical factors to develop a weight management plan to ensure success. For example, some owners may have concerns about the volume of food their pet can receive. In these instances, selecting a food with lower calorie density than the current diet may be appropriate to allow for a restriction of calories without decreasing the volume of food. This method helps avoid owner concern over satiety of the pet and minimizes attrition from weight management programs by addressing potential challenges proactively. Similarly, discussing the environment at home, such as the owner's work schedule, may also need to be integrated. For example, if a dog can only be taken out for a walk twice a day because of an owner's work schedule, a higher fiber diet that results in increased amount or more frequent fecal output may not be ideal for that environment. Needs of other pets in the household may also warrant consideration for similar logistics to ensure adherence. By understanding clients' backgrounds and perspectives, weight management, in particular, diet selection can be approached by the veterinarian in a way that clients will accept and engage in for optimal success.

SELECTING THE OPTIMAL NUTRIENT PROFILE

Once the veterinarian and owner agree that a pet's overweight or obese condition should be addressed, the specific diet plan must be designed. Owners often ask, "What is the best diet?" There really is no "best" diet for every overweight pet. There are several factors to consider before making a diet recommendation as part of a weight management plan, including those discussed above, and medical factors that will be discussed in this section.

The following recommendations assume an otherwise healthy overweight pet. For pets with comorbidities, additional nutritional modifications may be necessary. It is appropriate to contact a board-certified veterinary nutritionist for assistance with these more challenging weight loss cases.

Energy

Although the most fundamental aspect of a successful weight loss nutritional plan is to reduce calorie intake, simply feeding less of a pet's current diet is not necessarily an appropriate strategy.[10,11] Feeding less of the pet's diet may lead to food-seeking behaviors and leave the owner frustrated that the pet is hungry, while also increasing the risk of nutrient deficiency.[10] One key factor to consider when reducing energy intake is calorie density of the diet(s) to be fed.

Feeding a diet with reduced calorie density typically provides the pet a larger volume of food, with the same (or fewer) calories than the pet was previously consuming. This method leaves owners feeling that the pet is satiated and usually reduces begging behavior. It also allows for flexibility in decreasing volume fed later on when further nutrient and calorie reduction is required to maintain weight loss, as it minimizes concern of malnutrition or nutrient deficiency. Techniques to reduce calorie density often include added fiber (primarily insoluble fiber), water (canned food), or air (decreased kibble density).

Adult maintenance diets available over the counter (OTC) for cats and dogs vary widely in calorie density. Although there is not an extensive review of currently available diets, canine and feline maintenance dry kibble diets often range from 3500 to 4000 kcal/kg, and canned diets are approximately 1000 kcal/kg. According to the Association of American Feed Control Officials (AAFCO) regulations, a low-calorie, light, or lite diet must provide fewer than 3100 and 3250 kcal/kg, respectively, for canine and feline dry kibble diets or fewer than 900 and 950 kcal/kg, respectively, for canned diets.[12]

However, diets can be marketed for weight loss without using these terms, thus, not falling under this requirement, which causes confusion for pet owners. In addition, there are no volume restrictions under AAFCO guidelines, such as kilocalories per cup or per can, which is how most US pet owners measure pet food. One study reviewed all of the currently available diets marketed for weight management, including those with and without terms that fall under AAFCO's calorie restriction guidelines.[8] Therapeutic and OTC dry foods marketed for weight management ranged from 217 to 440 kcal/cup (for dogs) and 235 to 480 kcal/cup (for cats). Additionally, recommendations for feeding directions vary and are based on the pet's current weight, which in many cases leads to weight gain instead of loss.[8] Given these findings, recommendations for specific diets should be made, as vague directions to select a light food, which would lead to further confusion and possible weight gain, would be inappropriate. Currently, labeling for all complete and balanced diets for dogs and cats requires calorie density as kilocalorie per cup or can and kilocalorie per kilogram. This labeling may help veterinarians provide general guidance, such as recommending dry foods that provide approximately 300 kcal/cup and less than AAFCO guidelines of 3100 kcal/kg (dogs) and 3250 kcal/kg (cats) or canned foods that provide approximately 30 kcal/oz and less than the AAFCO guidelines of 900 kcal/kg (dogs) and 950 kcal/kg (cats).[12] These are starting calorie density guidelines based on successful management of clinical cases by the authors.

Macronutrients

In addition to calorie intake, it is important to consider the sources of those calories. Energy (calories) is derived from 3 macronutrients: protein, fat, and carbohydrates. Optimal proportion of these macronutrients for each pet should be considered when selecting a diet.

Protein

Ensuring adequate protein intake is imperative for the pet to maintain lean body mass (muscle).[13] Minimal recommendations for protein intake have been made to meet the National Research Council's recommended intake or minimal requirement (**Box 1, Table 1**).[14] Currently available veterinary therapeutic weight loss diets range from 8.4 to 13.0 and 10.5 to 13.8 g of protein per 100 kcal for dogs and cats, respectively. This example shows another time when a pet's potential comorbidities should be considered. For example, for an obese dog with protein-losing nephropathy, less protein than typically found in a veterinary therapeutic weight loss diet is indicated to provide adequate protein without exacerbating their clinical condition. Additionally, if any pet has a comorbidity that contradicts the preferred nutrient profile for weight loss (particularly increased levels of protein), consultation with a board-certified veterinary nutritionist is recommended to determine the optimal nutrient profile. Lastly, a

---

Box 1
Evaluating protein sufficiency using resting energy requirements and body weight

Because labels do not show protein content in grams per 1000 kcal, the grams of protein being fed can be calculated using the "guaranteed analysis" and the following information:

Assume an overweight dog with 10 kg ideal body weight. Assume your food label shows 21% crude protein and contains 3490 kcal/kg.

1. Calculate dog's caloric needs at 80% resting energy requirements (see text), use the following equation:

    $80\% \ (70 \times 10 \ kg^{0.75}) = 315 \ kcal/d$

2. Calculate grams of protein in the food using the following equation:

    (% crude protein/kcal/kg) × 10.000 = g/1000 kcal of food
    21/3.490 kcal/kg × 10.000 = 60 g/1000 kcal

3. Determine dog's daily protein requirement using the following equation:

    ≥5 g/kg for cats and 2.5 g/kg for dogs
    2.5 g/kg × 10 kg BW = 25 g/d protein

4. Determine whether the food provides sufficient protein to meet canine pet's needs using the following:

    315 kcal/d × 60 g/1000 kcal = 18.9 g/d
    18 g <25 g

This food does not provide sufficient protein.

From Brooks D, Churchill J, Fein K, et al. 2014 AAHA weight management guidelines for dogs and cats. J Am Anim Hosp Assoc 2014;50(1):1–11.

Table 1 Minimum protein requirements in diets		
	Minimum Protein Needed in Diet to Meet NRC Recommended Allowances	
NRC Recommended Allowances for Protein/kg of Ideal BW Per Day	When Fed at 80% of RER for Ideal BW	When Fed at 60% of RER for Ideal BW
Cat 4.96 g protein/BW (kg)$^{0.67}$	89 g/1000 kcal	104 g/1000 kcal
Dog 3.28 g protein/BW (kg)$^{0.75}$	60 g/1000 kcal	79 g/1000 kcal

Abbreviations: BW, body weight; NRC, National Research Council; RER, resting energy requirement.
From Brooks D, Churchill J, Fein K, et al. 2014 AAHA weight management guidelines for dogs and cats. J Am Anim Hosp Assoc 2014;50(1):1–11.

discussion should occur between the veterinarian, the owner, and any board-certified veterinary nutritionist consulted about whether weight loss is even appropriate and to what extent it would benefit or harm the pet, given the severity and type of comorbidities of the pet. In some disease conditions, although it is not helpful for the pet to be overweight before diagnosis of a disease, being overweight once a disease is diagnosed has been associated with increased survival times, deemed the obesity paradox. This paradox has been seen in renal disease and cardiac disease.[15,16] These cases should be reviewed carefully for what is in the best interest of the pet, given its specific condition.

Fat
There is a myth that low fat equates to low calorie. Although 1 g of fat does provide 2.25 times more calories than 1 g of protein or carbohydrates, this does not mean that all low-fat diets are appropriate for weight loss. Many veterinary therapeutic canine weight loss diets are reduced in fat, typically providing fewer than 3 g of fat per 100 kcal; however, it is possible for reduced-fat diets to provide significantly more calories than desired for a weight loss plan (eg, having a high calorie density in terms of kilocalories per kilogram or kilocalories per cup or can).

Carbohydrates
Another myth in veterinary medicine is that low-carbohydrate diets promote weight loss, particularly in cats. In humans, one alternative weight loss method is to induce a ketotic state by eliminating carbohydrate intake. However, it is not clear if this state can be induced in dogs and cats or if it is beneficial for weight loss in any species. In fact, veterinary studies have found that calorie intake, not carbohydrate intake, is associated with obesity.[17] Further, veterinary therapeutic low-carbohydrate diets designed for management of cats with diabetes mellitus can have very high calorie density, particularly in dry kibble diets, providing up to 500 to 600 kcal/cup. Depending on volume fed and owner adherence (owners may be resistant to feed a small volume because of the high calorie density), this diet may promote weight gain in overweight cats, even though some products are marketed for weight management.

Micronutrients
Micronutrients should be considered from multiple perspectives. In people, it is suggested that micronutrient deficiencies actually contribute to obesity.[18,19] The cause-effect relationship between obesity and micronutrient deficiency is unclear. Nonetheless, diet micronutrient concentrations should be considered when

formulating a weight loss plan. In people, intake of low-fat milk with supplemented micronutrients (iron, magnesium, vitamin E, niacin, thiamin, vitamin B-6, and vitamin B-12) as part of an energy-restricted diet, contributed to greater loss of body weight and body fat versus low-fat milk without micronutrients groups and control groups.[18]

Feeding a restricted number of calories from any diet may induce nutrient deficiencies if the nutrient/calorie ratio is insufficient. One study evaluated the risk for development of hypothetical nutrient deficiencies using different degrees of calorie restriction with 5 commercial canine diets of variable calorie density (2 veterinary therapeutic weight loss diets and 3 OTC diets).[10] Multiple nutrients were determined to be less than the National Research Council Recommended Allowance for adult maintenance at varying levels of energy restriction, including resting energy requirement for ideal weight. Selenium and choline were the nutrients calculated most likely to be deficient.[10] This study was ex vivo, and results cannot be directly extrapolated to pets undergoing weight loss; however, results do suggest that there is potential for micronutrient deficiencies to develop in pets undergoing extreme calorie restriction. This study supports the need for careful consideration of nutrient/calorie ratios, with increasing scrutiny as calorie restriction intensifies. Two further in vivo studies showed a lack of clinical signs when participants were fed purpose-formulated weight management diets in a clinical setting.[20,21] These findings cannot be extrapolated to show that all veterinary therapeutic weight loss diets will not cause deficiency, but it suggests that there may be less inherent risk for nutrient deficiency with a purpose-formulated diet for weight loss as opposed to feeding less of an adult maintenance diet. The optimal micronutrient profile for weight management is still unknown, although recent American Animal Hospital Association (AAHA) Weight Management Guidelines recommend consulting a board-certified veterinary nutritionist for cases that require fewer than 60% of resting energy requirements for ideal weight to ensure adequate diet formulation.[14]

Additional Diet Factors

Fiber
Additional diet factors may influence weight loss in dogs and cats. Fiber is often touted as a nutrient that contributes to successful weight loss. To understand potential benefits, fiber should be considered for its solubility and fermentability properties. Diets high in insoluble fiber (eg, cellulose, hemicellulose) are typically lower in calorie density and allow pets to eat a greater volume of food, although these can increase fecal output. Diets containing fermentable fibers that result in short-chain fatty acid production may influence satiety by increasing concentrations of satiety-inducing gastrointestinal hormones, peripheral peptide tyrosine-tyrosine and glucagonlike peptide 1.[22] In one study, a high-protein, high-fiber diet had a greater influence on satiety in healthy dogs than either a high-protein or high-fiber diet.[23] Nonetheless, other studies found no impact of higher fiber content.[24,25] A diet history and nutritional assessment will guide the amount of fiber that should be considered for each pet.

Water
Increasing water concentration of a diet may also aid in weight loss. Voluntary energy intake and body weight decreased in cats fed a canned diet with higher water content than a freeze-dried version of the same diet.[26] Anecdotally, some clients report that increasing water concentration helps their pets feel more satiated. However, this method may be cost-prohibitive in larger pets. If dry food is being fed, an owner could consider adding water to the kibble if the pet tolerates it.

Other additives

The addition of certain food additives (eg, L-carnitine, α-lipoic acid, betaine) is recommended by some to improve fatty acid metabolism and increase lean body mass during weight loss in cats and rats.[27,28] Ultimately, although there may be some beneficial effects with the use of these additives, more evidence is necessary before widespread use is warranted. Calorie restriction using an appropriate weight loss diet remains the hallmark of a successful weight loss program.

EVIDENCE-BASED SELECTION OF DIETS

Many factors, both medical and pet driven or owner driven, should be considered when selecting a weight loss diet. The optimal nutrient profile should be determined by detailed diet history, physical examination, and nutritional assessment. Based on that predetermined nutrient profile, a diet should then be selected that meets that nutrient profile. An algorithm is included to assist in developing a nutrient profile for each pet (**Fig. 1**).

ENERGY RESTRICTION
Initial Calculation

As discussed in the previous sections, obtaining an accurate diet history allows for an accurate estimation of daily calorie intake, and a 10% to 20% reduction in that calorie amount is a reasonable starting point for daily calorie intake in a weight loss plan. If that is not possible, feeding the resting energy requirement (RER = 70 x body weight $[BW]_{kg}^{0.75}$) for the pet's estimated ideal body weight is one of many other options.[4] For pets weighing 2 to 25 kg, a linear equation can be used: (RER = $30 \times BW_{kg} + 70$); however, this equation will overestimate calorie needs for larger pets. Regardless of which calculation is used, it is important to realize that this is just a starting point; some overweight pets may already be eating close to those calculated amounts, and further calorie restriction will be required to achieve weight loss. If further adjustment is needed, the optimal diet for each pet may change, so frequent assessment of weight management cases is essential to meet the changing nutrient needs of the pet.

Rate of Weight Loss

The target rate of weight loss depends on each pet and their unique circumstances. Rates of successful weight loss range from 0.5% to 2% of weekly body weight loss for cats and dogs.[14] Different rates of weight loss may provide additional benefits, with one study showing 1% of body weight loss per week limited risk of nutrient deficiency, loss of lean body mass, and rebound weight gain.[13] The nutritional assessment of the pet and the initial discussion with the owner often guides the rate of weight loss. Using the readiness to change scale and asking owners whether they prefer to see quicker results (and thus a more aggressive rate of weight loss) or whether they prefer to have slow gradual change (which would steer the plan toward a smaller rate of weight loss) will increase adherence to the selected plan. Although some owners may need to see faster results to minimize attrition, others may want to cease weight management plans if they feel their pet is losing weight too fast and experiencing behaviors they attribute to hunger owing to the more aggressive weight loss. With these considerations, individualization and frequent adjustment is essential to optimal adherence.

Exceptions include pets with comorbidities in which a more gradual rate of loss (0.5% or less) is recommended, although further studies are needed to determine target rates in various disease conditions or whether weight loss is indicated at all

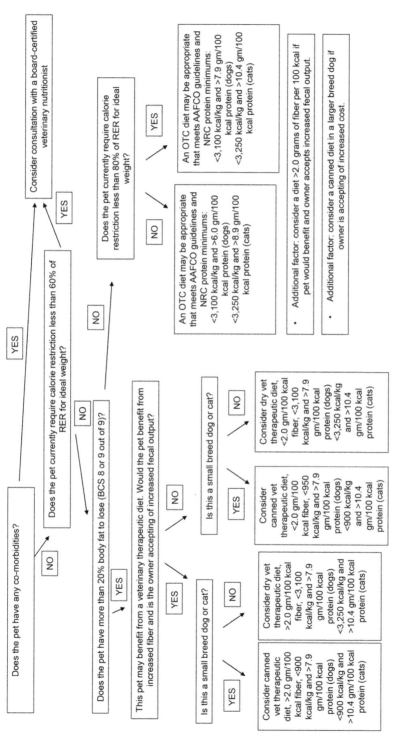

Fig. 1. Algorithm to select a weight loss diet.

in certain diseases. Additionally, cats and dogs may subsequently have decreased energy requirements when faced with calorie restriction.[29] When severe calorie restriction is necessary (less than 60% resting energy requirement for ideal weight), it is critical to ensure appropriate diet selection to provide adequate essential nutrients and to prepare owners that further restriction may be necessary. At this level of restriction, a board-certified veterinary nutritionist should be consulted to ensure optimal nutrient profile selection, or possible supplementation, even with veterinary therapeutic diets.

Commonly, pets' weight plateaus during their weight loss. When this occurs, it is recommended to reduce the calorie intake by approximately 10% and increase physical activity if possible. Measuring the food by weight (ie, in grams on a kitchen scale), can allow for more precise adjustments. Successful weight loss plans may take up to 1 year or more and require close contact with owners to help them make adjustments as needed to avoid frustration and failure. At every check in, the rate of weight loss and diet selection should be reviewed and discussed with the owner. The needs of the pet and the owner may change over time and require adjustment, so frequent and consistent assessment can proactively address challenges and barriers to successful weight loss.

MAINTENANCE OF WEIGHT LOSS

Once a pet reaches ideal body weight, unfortunately calorie intake often does not increase to maintain that healthy weight. For many, it is best to continue feeding the diet fed during the weight loss at the same amount (if at a plateau) or to increase calorie intake by approximately 5%. Another discussion similar to the initial assessment can determine if a pet owner wants to pursue this method or if they prefer to transition to another diet, potentially an OTC maintenance diet if a veterinary therapeutic weight loss diet was previously used. Even though the goal is not active weight loss, the level of calorie restriction should guide selection of the optimal diet (see **Fig. 1**). Careful diet selection for maintenance is just as critical as it is during active weight loss to avoid the weight gain that can occur by switching to a maintenance diet. Unfortunately, reinduction of excess weight occurs much more easily with pets that have previously been overweight,[29] so lifelong monitoring of calorie intake is required, and owners should be counseled on lifelong management of their pet's weight.

STRATEGIES FOR INCREASED DIET ADHERENCE

An important component of successful weight management is the role that human–pet relationships can play in affecting obesity treatment and adherence to diet management. Owners may need social and psychological support in addition to veterinary medical support to achieve diet adherence and improve success in weight management. Aspects of the human–pet bond can, therefore, be integrated into the diet plan to improve owner satisfaction and ability to implement the diet plan recommended. Treats, physical activity, resources available for the veterinary health care team to use to increase adherence, and the relevance of these aspects to diet management will be addressed.

Treats and Non-negotiables

Providing treats is central to many pet owners' relationships with their pets, especially in dogs. One survey study of pet owners found that they were willing to engage in veterinary guidance, adhere to diet modification, use a veterinary weight loss product, increase exercise, and attend an obesity clinic to get their pet to lose weight before they considered eliminating treats.[30] Incorporating treats into the diet plan can preserve the pet–owner relationship without compromising weight loss. A discussion about treats should occur during the diet history and again while considering the optimal diet. Some owners may wish to simplify the plan and not provide treats, but most will likely need this as a part of their plan. For those owners, it is helpful to discuss compromise and limit all food items that are not complete and balanced to less than 10% of the total calorie intake. This action requires the veterinary health care team to calculate the total recommended diet intake and then subtract 10% for treats while determining what amount of the main diet would compromise 90% of that calorie amount. For example, a daily feeding schedule could be discussed for a 35-kg pet that included 1000 kcal total (resting energy requirement for ideal weight) with 900 kcal in a therapeutic weight loss food and 10% of the total 1000 kcal (100 kcal) reserved for favorite treats.

Non-negotiables can be included in this treat allowance, including food items that may be over the allowance, which would then take up more than 1 days' allowance (eg, if a daily treat allowance for a dog was 100 kcal, but a favorite treat that the owners feel they cannot remove from the regimen is a 200-kcal chew treat, then that would be the only items outside the main diet that pet can receive for 2 days). This adjustment allows owners to feel comforted that the veterinary health care team respects their relationship with their pet and that they don't need to choose between what they feel is depriving their pet of their love and keeping them healthy. Some examples of low-calorie treats include nonstarch vegetables such as carrots or celery. As an alternative, small portions of the daily allotment of food can be given throughout the day as treats. Incorporating favorite treats into the diet plan can alleviate some owner's concerns about feared rigidity of weight loss programs, perceived lack of palatability in weight loss diets, and concern of deprivation of the pet (many of these concerns come from pet owners' experiences with weight loss in themselves or in human medicine in general). This method allows for flexibility and creativity on the owners' part to ensure they are able to provide their pet with something they love and thus maintain a strong human–pet bond, which is so often linked to providing favored food items.

Troubleshooting and Addressing Client Concerns

When collecting a diet history and discussing the diet plan, owners should also be asked about their relationship with their pet and what potential challenges they foresee. This information may help the veterinarian develop a weight management plan that capitalizes on the owner–pet relationship that already exists. In addition, in-depth knowledge of the pet–owner relationship helps identify and preemptively address any potential barriers to weight management plan adherence. For example, discussing potential concerns from owners about cost or common myths and misconceptions (eg, incorrectly assuming fiber is a filler with no benefit to the pet) before engaging in the weight management program can help guide diet plans or troubleshooting when issues arise. For troubleshooting on a variety of common challenges, the AAHA Weight Management Guidelines provide tips and tricks for veterinarians that range from managing begging behavior to a pet not accepting a new diet.[14] Because weight management plans can be rather labor intensive, veterinarians can use as many premade resources as possible, such as frequently asked question handouts on nutrition-related myths or owner-directed guides for selecting pet foods. A list of these resources can be found in **Box 2**.

SUMMARY/DISCUSSION

Optimal diet selection is based on gathering as much pertinent information as possible from a diet history, nutritional assessment, and in-depth discussion with pet owners to determine the needs of the pet and the environment in which the pet lives. Many factors, such as medical needs of the pet and aspects that impact the human–pet bond, can guide selection of a nutrient profile that will ensure successful weight management. Careful consideration of calorie density, macronutrients, micronutrients, and owner preferences will minimize risk of nutrient deficiency and unwanted begging behaviors or attrition from weight loss programs. Consistent and frequent monitoring of pets undergoing weight management allows for careful and appropriate adjustment of the plan not only during active weight loss but for successful lifelong management of a healthier pet at ideal weight.

REFERENCES

1. Laflamme D. Development and validation of a body condition score system for dogs. A clinical tool. Canine Pract 1997;22:10–5.
2. Laflamme D. Development and validation of a body condition score system for cats. A clinical tool. Feline Pract 1997;25:13–8.
3. Michel KE, Anderson W, Cupp C, et al. Correlation of a feline muscle mass score with body composition determined by dual-energy X-ray absorptiometry. Br J Nutr 2011;106(S1):S57–9.
4. Baldwin K, Bartges J, Buffington T, et al. AAHA nutritional assessment guidelines for dogs and cats. J Am Anim Hosp Assoc 2010;46(4):285–96.
5. Freeman L, Becvarova I, Cave N, et al. WSAVA nutritional assessment guidelines. Compend Contin Educ Vet 2011;33(8):E1–9.
6. Sapowicz S, Freeman LM, Linder DE. Body condition scores and evaluation of feeding habits of dogs and cats at a low cost veterinary clinic and a general practice. Presented in abstract form at 2014 American Academy of Veterinary Nutrition Symposium. Nashville (TN), June 4, 2014.
7. Churchill J. Increase the success of weight loss programs by creating an environment for change. Compend Contin Educ Vet 2010;32(12):E1.

8. Linder DE, Freeman LM. Evaluation of calorie density and feeding directions for commercially available diets designed for weight loss in cats and dogs. J Am Vet Med Assoc 2010;236(1):74–7.

9. Linder DE, Mueller MK. Pet obesity management: beyond nutrition. Vet Clin North Am Small Anim Pract 2014;44(4):789–806.

10. Linder DE, Freeman LM, Morris P, et al. Theoretical evaluation of risk for nutritional deficiency with caloric restriction in dogs. Vet Q 2012;32(3–4):123–9.

11. Linder DE, Freeman LM, Holden SL, et al. Status of selected nutrients in obese dogs undergoing caloric restriction. BMC Vet Res 2013;9:219.

12. Association of American Feed Control Officials Official Publication. Association of American Feed Control Officials. 2015. Available at: www.aafco.org. Accessed January 20, 2016.

13. Laflamme DP, Hannah SS. Increased diet protein promotes fat loss and reduces loss of lean body mass during weight loss in cats. Int J Appl Res Vet Med 2005; 3(2):62–8.

14. Brooks D, Churchill J, Fein K, et al. 2014 AAHA weight management guidelines for dogs and cats. J Am Anim Hosp Assoc 2014;50(1):1–11.

15. Slupe JL, Freeman LM, Rush JE. Association of body weight and body condition with survival in dogs with heart failure. J Vet Intern Med 2008;22(3):561–5.

16. Parker VJ, Freeman LM. Association between body condition and survival in dogs with acquired chronic kidney disease. J Vet Intern Med 2011;25(6):1306–11.

17. Backus RC, Cave NJ, Keisler DH. Gonadectomy and high diet fat but not high diet carbohydrate induce gains in body weight and fat of domestic cats. Br J Nutr 2007;98(3):641–50.

18. Rosado JL, Garcia OP, Ronquillo D, et al. Intake of milk with added micronutrients increases the effectiveness of an energy-restricted diet to reduce body weight: a randomized controlled clinical trial in Mexican women. J Am Diet Assoc 2011; 111:1507–16.

19. Garcia OP, Long KZ, Rosado JL. Impact of micronutrient deficiencies on obesity. Nutr Rev 2009;67(10):559–72.

20. German AJ, Holden SL, Serisier S, et al. Assessing the adequacy of essential nutrient intake in obese dogs undergoing energy restriction for weight loss: a cohort study. BMC Vet Res 2015;11:253.

21. German AJ, Titcomb JM, Holden SL, et al. Cohort study of the success of controlled weight loss programs for obese dogs. J Vet Intern Med 2015;29(6):1547–55.

22. Bosch G, Verbrugghe A, Hesta M, et al. The effects of diet fibre type on satiety-related hormones and voluntary food intake in dogs. Br J Nutr 2009;102:318–25.

23. Weber M, Bissot T, Servet E, et al. A high-protein, high-fiber diet designed for weight loss improves satiety in dogs. J Vet Intern Med 2007;21(6):1203–8.

24. Butterwick RF, Hawthorne AJ. Advances in diet management of obesity in dogs and cats. J Nutr 1998;128(12S):2771S–5S.

25. Yamka RM, Frantz NZ, Friesen KG. Effects of three canine weight loss foods on body composition and obesity markers. Int J Appl Res Vet Med 2007;5(3):125–32.

26. Wei A, Fascetti AJ, Villaverde C, et al. Effect of water content in a canned food on voluntary food intake and body weight in cats. Am J Vet Res 2011;72(7):918–23.

27. Center SA, Warner KL, Randolph JF, et al. Influence of diet supplementation with L-carnitine on metabolic rate, fatty acid oxidation, body condition, and weight loss in overweight cats. Am J Vet Res 2012;73(7):1002–15.

28. Jang A, Kim D, Sung KS, et al. The effect of diet α-lipoic acid, betaine, L-carnitine, and swimming on the obesity of mice induced by a high-fat diet. Food Funct 2014;5:1966–74.

29. Nagaoka D, Mitsuhashi Y, Angell R, et al. Re-induction of obese body weight occurs more rapidly and at lower caloric intake in beagles. J Anim Physiol Anim Nutr (Berl) 2010;94(3):287–92.

30. Bland IM, Guthrie-Jones A, Taylor RD, et al. Dog obesity: veterinary practices' and owners' opinions on cause and management. Prev Vet Med 2010;94(3–4): 310–5.

Obesity Treatment
Environment and Behavior Modification

 CrossMark

Maryanne Murphy, DVM, PhD

KEYWORDS

- Obesity • Weight management • Canine • Feline • Behavior • Environment
- Exercise • 5 A's

KEY POINTS

- Engage pet owners in planning sessions to determine feeding strategies they can realistically use in their home in order to improve owner adherence to diet recommendations.
- With adjustments for individual pet and owner ability, weight loss plans should include walking 3 times daily for a total of 30 to 45 minutes per day.
- Consider pointed behavior control strategies (eg, temptation resistance, temptation prevention, strict commitment, commitment by punishment, self-affirmation, and implementation intentions) with particular application to the owner.
- Consider use of the 5 A's behavioral counseling approach to recommend realistic plans from the initial consultation and adjust those plans throughout the weight loss phase.

INTRODUCTION

Obesity is commonly encountered in veterinary patients, with up to 59% of dogs[1–13] and up to 63% of cats[10,14–24] throughout the world classified as overweight or obese. Although many have documented approaches to induce weight loss in these veterinary patients,[25–33] successful long-term prevention of weight regain has proven elusive.[34–37] Similar results have been found in people,[38–40] and physiologic alterations in energy homeostatic mechanisms immediately after weight loss have been implicated as a cause of weight regain.[41] Exposure to an "obesogenic" environment with pervasive marketing and easily accessible large portions of energy-dense foods, stress-induced food consumption, and decreased physical activity makes maintenance of a healthy body mass index (BMI) difficult.[42] Individual sustained behavior modification is also a factor in prevention of weight gain with self-monitoring of intake, advance meal planning, use of lower calorie foods, regular weight checks, promoting self-efficacy, goal-setting, and problem-solving found to be effective.[42,43]

The author has nothing to disclose.
Department of Clinical Nutrition, Red Bank Veterinary Hospital, 197 Hance Avenue, Tinton Falls, NJ 07724, USA
E-mail address: murphvet@gmail.com

Vet Clin Small Anim 46 (2016) 883–898
http://dx.doi.org/10.1016/j.cvsm.2016.04.009   **vetsmall.theclinics.com**

Although the pet is the primary concern of the veterinary team, any proposed weight management strategy for obesity must take the pet's owner into consideration.[44–47] Because the owner directly affects the environment and behavior of the pet, treatment strategies with a focus on owner involvement are the focus of this review. Dietary strategies to induce weight loss in cats and dogs have been reviewed elsewhere (see Deborah E. Linder and Valerie J. Parker's article, "Dietary Aspects of Weight Management in Cats and Dogs," in this issue).[32,45,48]

ENVIRONMENT SPECIFIC TREATMENT
Feeding Management

An important environmental factor in obesity is the way the pet is being fed. Ad libitum feeding has been identified as a risk factor for cat obesity in some studies,[17,49,50] but not in others.[14,16,18,20,23] Meal frequency in cats or dogs is inconsistently associated with obesity risk.[2,4,8,15,16,21,51] Provision of treats, table scraps, or other homemade foods has been associated with an increased risk of overweight or obesity,[2,5–8,12,50,51] although not always.[15,52] Despite the inconsistencies, use of measured amounts fed individually as scheduled meals is recommended during weight loss plans to control total daily energy intake.[25,26,48,53–55] The owner should be engaged in a planning session in order to find a solution the owner can reasonably implement while following the prescribed recommendations regarding appropriate total energy intake for their pet.

Separation of pets during meal times via kennels (**Fig. 1**), baby gates, microchip feeders, controlled monitoring, elevated feedings, and so forth should be considered as part of a discrete, consistent routine. When diverting from previous norms is challenging, household members may work on gradually changing both their and their pet's behaviors.[53] Habituate animals with free access to food to free access during scheduled parts of the day with eventual transition to isolated meal feeding. Cats exhibit increased appetitive behaviors and affection when exposed to caloric restriction but no behavioral difference with reduction from ad libitum versus habituated meal feeding.[56] Owners of obese dogs tend to interpret every need as a request for food,[57]

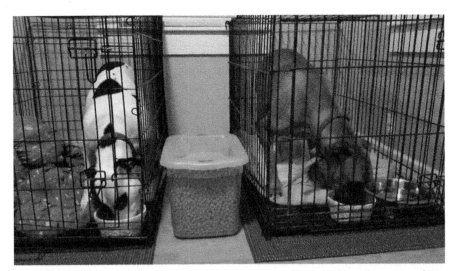

Fig. 1. Dogs fed in separate kennels to inhibit access to each other's food. (*Courtesy of* Maryanne Murphy, DVM, PhD, Tinton Falls, NJ.)

and owners of obese cats give in more frequently to begging behavior.[50] Owners should limit pet access to food preparation and consumption areas of the home; this may serve as an opportunity to simultaneously feed the pet its own meal in a separate area to reduce excess feeding temptation. Pet owners should be advised to use smaller bowls and serving scoops to reduce the volume of food portioned[58] or weigh out daily food offerings to improve precision and accuracy.[54]

Activity

Exercise and general activity level within the home environment should be modified as well. Reduced activity is associated with an increased obesity risk,[2,6,8,14,16,51] and risk of obesity in dogs decreases for every hour of weekly exercise.[2,6] Lean dogs spend significantly more time in vigorous daily activity compared with obese dogs,[59] and dog body condition score (BCS) is inversely related to number of steps taken per day.[60,61] In dogs undergoing weight loss, every 1000 steps taken allowed 1 kcal/kg$^{0.75}$ additional energy consumption while maintaining a weight loss rate of 2% per week.[27] Although data regarding optimal activity types for weight loss in cats and dogs are limited, enhanced weight loss via diet plans that include underwater treadmill and/or leash walking has been suggested.[62,63] To date, a single study has shown treadmill/leash-based activity maintains lean body mass in dogs during weight loss versus diet alone.[28] Continued leash walking after successful weight loss is recommended because spontaneous activity level in dogs does not increase while losing weight.[64]

Although these data support the use of exercise in weight loss plans, specific duration and intensity recommendations for optimal programs in cats and dogs do not yet exist. The 2014 American Animal Hospital Association Weight Management Guidelines for Dogs and Cats suggest a dog with no orthopedic restrictions should be walked for 5 minutes 3 times per day with an eventual increase to 30 to 45 minutes of total walking time per day, or up to the owner's or pet's limitations.[32] Activity level considerations for cats typically center on use of indoor environmental enrichment,[32,65] but the author has had owners leash walk cats during weight loss plans (**Fig. 2**). For successful implementation, recommendations must be tailored to the individual case. Owners may find recommendations to suddenly take 3 walks per day insurmountable and therefore be less likely to leash walk the pet at all. Regardless of the specific activity, the owner should document duration and frequency for accountability and to allow for adjustment throughout the weight loss plan.[32]

BEHAVIOR SPECIFIC TREATMENT

In addition to obesity management techniques focusing on the physical environment, the behavior of both the pet and the owner must also be addressed. Energy intake is influenced by homeostatic (driven by lack of energy intake) and reward-based (influenced by food palatability) neurobehavioral systems.[66,67] Within the reward-based system are the concepts of "liking" the sensory pleasure of eating the highly palatable food source and "wanting" to enjoy the liking sensation again.[66] Wanting can contribute to overconsumption because the neurobehavioral drive for reward has greater control over intake versus the homeostatic system.[67]

Although the "liking" and "wanting" sensations likely drive many begging behaviors exhibited by cats and dogs, owners often misinterpret these behaviors.[57] Pet animals are not capable of satisfying neurobehavioral cravings without help from their owners,

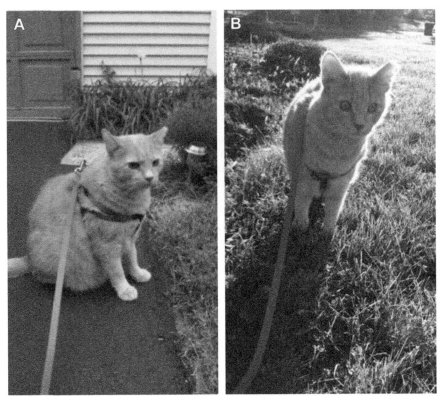

Fig. 2. Cat being leash walked during weight loss plan. (*A*) With initial exposure to the harness, Buddy spent most time sitting and observing. (*B*) After repeated use of the harness, Buddy began exploring the area and participating in daily leash walks. (*Courtesy of* Susan Vernosky, BBA, Eatontown, NJ.)

which is why the veterinary team, as part of the pet's weight loss plan, should consider owner specific behavior-control strategies. Strategies for weight loss are as follows[66]:

1. *Temptation resistance:* use willpower to ignore or inhibit cravings (eg, walk away when the pet is actively begging for food)
2. *Temptation prevention:* identify and then avoid environmental triggers of temptation (eg, limit pet access to food preparation and consumption areas of the home if the pet is habituated to receiving table scraps)
3. *Strict commitment:* limit future choices to more valuable, delayed rewards (eg, enroll the pet in an inpatient weight loss program to limit an owner's temptation to overfeed and allow for successful weight loss in the pet)
4. *Commitment by punishment:* identify a form of punishment to deter temptation at the point of decision (eg, make a predetermined financial contribution to a charitable fund when the pet's weight loss goal is not achieved at each recheck)

Although consideration of their implementation with behavioral management of the obese state is recommended, use of these strategies in the veterinary setting has not been investigated, and their specific utility in human weight loss plans needs further investigation.[68]

Pet owners may overfeed due to problems with goal setting, monitoring food intake and its impact, and acting as needed.[69] Use of self-affirmation and implementation intentions

---

Box 1
Behavior specific terms explained

- Self-affirmation: an act that maintains and protects a personal sense of self-integrity. Reflecting on self-affirmations can help remind the pet owner they have integrity and still have the best interests of their pet in mind.[70,71]
  - I am able to provide my pet with a safe home.
  - I love my pet and want to provide it the best quality of life.
  - I am able to provide toys to encourage activity for my pet.
  - I can take great care of my pet and provide it an environment to encourage weight loss.

- Implementation intention: a planning process to identify potential problems and solutions to determine situational responses before occurrence.[69,73,74]
  - If my pet begs for food, then I will purchase and use a portion-controlled automatic feeder.
  - If my pet sits near me when eating my own meals, then I will remove it from the kitchen while I eat.
  - If my pet is acting hungry, but it is not time to be fed, then I will take it for a walk or engage it in a playful activity.
  - If my pet gains access to food sitting on my kitchen counter, then I will place the food in a closed cabinet the pet cannot open.

- Self-concordance: ensure a goal reflects personal interests and values rather than something one feels compelled to do by other pressures.[75] The recommendations of the veterinary team may be more successful if the owner has an intrinsic reason to achieve the goal.
  - A pet owner who enjoys taking the pet for leash walks may be more likely to follow the frequency and duration of activity recommendations.
  - A pet owner interested in pursuing active weight loss for their pet may be more likely to follow diet and activity recommendations.
  - A pet owner excited about finding new combinations of treats to maintain within a daily recommended allowance will be more likely to reduce the total volume of daily treats as directed.

(if-then planning; **Box 1**) strategies to improve owner-related adherence to the prescribed weight loss plan can be considered. Self-affirmation describes the need to maintain and protect a personal sense of self-integrity in the face of threat to that integrity.[70,71] For an owner of an obese pet, their sense of self-integrity may be threatened when they realize their own behavior was a primary contributor to their pet's current health condition. Maintain the owner's individual valued identity with a self-affirmation demonstrating adequacy as a pet owner.[70,72] Owners may complete a self-affirmation exercise while waiting for their appointment or the veterinary team can use simple conversation to identify potential self-affirmations.[69] Ask the owner to identify ways in which they positively contribute to their pet's well-being (eg, able to provide the pet with a safe home, love the pet and want to provide them the best quality of life). This focus on the owner's self-worth may make them more receptive to continuing with the weight loss plan despite any setbacks.

Implementation intentions identify potential problems and solutions to determine situational responses before occurrence.[69,73,74] For example, if the cat wakes the owner up in the middle of the night to be fed, then the owner will purchase and use a portion-controlled automatic feeder. Intentions can be identified during veterinary appointments, but the owner should make adjustments as needed to maintain relevance within their own home. The intentions should reflect a state of self-concordance in which they signify the personal interests and feelings of the owner and are not influenced by external pressures from the veterinary team (see **Box 1**).[75] Employment of self-concordance improves successful implementation intention progress,[75–78] but is inhibited in those with self-critical tendencies.[79] A larger impact of intention success, however, comes from accessibility of the plan components.[80] An intention to use an automatic feeder is only successful if financially attainable. Failure to fully implement this intention may be due to financial constraints, not an issue with self-concordance. With medium- and long-term weight control, successful outcomes have been found in people with high levels of self-motivation, self-efficacy, self-regulation skills, flexible eating restraint, and positive body image.[81] Similar trends may exist with owners of overweight or obese pets, but further investigation is needed.

Effective Use of Behavior-Specific Treatments

Volitional help sheets aid people in the process of forming their own implementation intentions.[82] An obesity-specific sheet (**Table 1**) has been designed and was

Table 1
Volitional help sheet for weight loss

We want you to plan to lose weight. Research shows that if people can spot situations in which they will be tempted to eat and then link them with a way to overcome those situations, they are much more likely to be successful in losing weight. On the left hand side of the page below is a list of common situations in which people feel tempted to eat; on the right hand side of the page is a list of possible solutions. For each situation that applies to you personally (left hand side), please draw a line linking it to a solution (right hand side) that you think might work for you. Please draw a line linking one situation to one solution at a time, but make as many (or as few) situation-solution links as you like.

Situations	Solutions
☐ If I am tempted to eat when I am anxious.	☐ Then I will read about people who have successfully lost weight.
☐ If I am tempted to eat when I am depressed (or down).	☐ Then I will consider the belief that people who lose weight will help to improve the world.
☐ If I am tempted to eat when there are many different kinds of food available.	☐ Then I will leave places where people are eating a lot.
☐ If I am tempted to eat when I am at a party.	☐ Then I will be the object of discrimination because of my being overweight.
☐ If I am tempted to eat when I have to say "no" to others.	☐ Then I will I have someone who listens when I need to talk about my losing weight.
☐ If I am tempted to eat when I feel it's impolite to refuse a second helping.	☐ Then I will take diet pills to help me lose weight.
☐ If I am tempted to eat when others are pressuring me to eat.	☐ Then I will reward myself when I do not overeat.
☐ If I am tempted to eat when I have a headache.	☐ Then I will tell myself that if I try hard enough I can keep from overeating.
☐ If I am tempted to eat when I feel uncomfortable.	☐ Then I will do something else instead of eating when I need to relax or deal with tension.
☐ If I am tempted to eat when I am watching TV.	☐ Then I will remember studies about illnesses caused by being overweight that have upset me.
☐ If I am tempted to eat just before going to bed.	☐ Then I will struggle to alter my view of myself as an overweight person.
☐ If I am tempted to eat when I am happy.	☐ Then I will remove things from my home that remind me of eating.

From Armitage CJ, Norman P, Noor M, et al. Evidence that a very brief psychological intervention boosts weight loss in a weight loss program. Behav Ther 2014;45(5):706; with permission.

associated with enhanced weight loss compared with people participating in a controlled weight loss program alone.[83] Until a veterinary-specific sheet is developed and validated, the owner should identify and document personally relevant situations and the responses they think will help.[69] Use of a standard form will improve appointment efficiency and provide a framework for plan modification during subsequent visits. As the weight loss plan progresses, owners should review these situations and self-report their actual responses during the time since the last visit.[69]

Maximizing Weight Loss Success with the 5 A's Behavioral Counseling Approach

In human medicine, various clinical practice guidelines designed to improve individual aspects of patients' health have been developed, but successful implementation into clinical practice is often slow.[84] With a specific goal of aiding guideline adoption, a consistent behavioral counseling approach used to modify risky behaviors across clinical care has been developed. This Five A's system, as outlined by the Canadian Task Force on Preventive Care, and adopted by the US Preventive Services Task Force of the Agency for Healthcare Research and Quality, is as follows[85]:

1. *Assess:* ask about health risks and any factors affecting choice of behavior change suggestions
2. *Advise:* give specific information about why the behavior is considered risky
3. *Agree:* collaborate to ensure both interest and willingness on the patient's part to change the behavior
4. *Assist:* use specific behavior change techniques to help the patient succeed and supplement with adjunctive medical therapy as indicated
5. *Arrange:* aid in scheduling of treatment referrals, provide follow-up contact to ensure patient adherence, adjust the treatment plan as needed

When specifically applied to obesity management in human beings, the 5 A's guide the physician from initial diagnosis and conversation with the individual to final arrangement of outside expert referral if warranted.[85–87] For veterinarians treating or preventing obesity in canine and feline patients, it is proposed that this behavioral modification construct is applicable when aiming for behavioral change on the part of the pet owner (**Fig. 3**). Pet owners should be considered part of the weight loss plan because they have been viewed as a main cause of pet obesity due to their role in the diet, socioeconomic status, and activity level within the pet's home.[2,4,6,16,18,21,51,57,88,89] The owner acts as the patient in the veterinary application of the 5 A's because the owner is responsible for doing the work of change.[87] These tactics may especially resonate with owners of obese dogs because the degree to which the dog is overweight has been correlated to the BMI of the dog owner.[7,57,90]

Use of the 5 A's in Veterinary Obesity Management

The primary veterinarian must first *assess* the cat or dog as being obese (BCS $\geq$ 8/9)[32] or as overweight (BCS 6 to 7/9). The pet's BCS should be documented as representative of an ideal, target, overweight, or obese weight. An ideal weight represents an animal with optimal body mass, whereas a target weight is a value determined to be appropriate for that pet by the clinician. The target weight may equal the ideal weight or it may provide allowances for animals with which reduction to ideal weight is deemed inappropriate.[91] If comorbidities known to interfere with successful weight loss (eg, hypothyroidism, hyperadrenocorticism, diabetes mellitus)[5] exist, appropriate treatment should be performed concurrently with the weight loss plan.

The veterinarian should address BCS with the owner at each interaction and *advise* weight adjustment as appropriate. If weight maintenance is appropriate, the owner

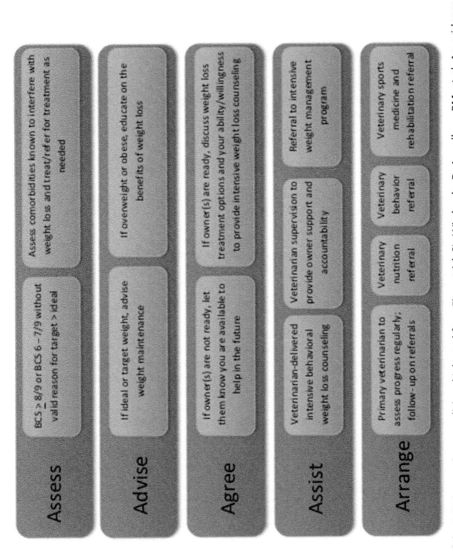

Fig. 3. Proposed use of the 5 A's in veterinary medicine. (*Adapted from* Fitzpatrick SL, Wischenka D, Appelhans BM, et al. An evidence-based guide for obesity treatment in primary care. Am J Med 2016;129(1):115.e3; with permission.)

should be advised of this to better ensure the current BCS is sustained. If weight loss is necessary, the owner should be educated on the benefits (eg, prolonged lifespan,[92] improved lameness with osteoarthritis,[93–95] improved insulin sensitivity[96,97]). When the owner understands the risks associated with obesity, improved motivation to make necessary changes may follow.[86] In one study, owner education did not affect the success of a weight loss plan.[98] However, a second study, looking into the effect of obese dog feeding practices before weight loss, found limited effect of prior feeding practices on the outcome of the weight loss plan. The investigators concluded owner education provided during the weight loss phase may have been responsible for changing prior habits and practices, thus allowing successful weight loss.[99]

Once educated, the owner should be asked to *agree* with the plan. If agreement is not achieved, the veterinarian should offer to be of assistance when the owner is ready. Weight loss should be readdressed at the next opportunity to determine if the owner has become agreeable to change. When agreement is achieved, it is suggested to create specific, measureable, attainable, relevant, and time-based (SMART) goals to aid behavioral counseling success.[86,87,100] These goals are another form of directed problem solving similar to implementation intentions described earlier. A veterinary-specific example is, "I will feed my pet 30 Calories of treats every day of the week," as opposed to, "I will feed my pet less treats." Whenever the owner mentions a vague goal, such as, "I will reduce my dog's access to the cat's food," the veterinarian can develop the SMART goal as, "I will place my cat's food bowl on the top perch of the cat tree every day since the dog cannot reach that surface." These updated goals can be written down to allow for easy owner reference and adherence at home. If the veterinarian is not able or willing to help the owner with this step, referral for advanced weight loss plan development is appropriate.

Assisting the owner as the plan is implemented is the fourth construct of the 5 A's. The veterinarian who recommended weight loss and made initial feeding recommendations should be available for pet and owner follow-up. The veterinary team is tasked not only with support when a weight loss plateau occurs or when the owner struggles with ignoring the pet's begging for additional food but also with being a source of accountability. Any barriers to achieving the SMART goals or implementation intentions generated during the agreement step can be addressed by developing pointed strategies to overcome the barriers.[86,87] This assistance phase is another opportunity to consider specialty referral, especially if the primary veterinary team or the owner becomes discouraged by a lack of perceived success or compliance.

If specialty referral is made, the veterinary team should be heavily involved in ease of its *arrangement*. A staff member may call the referral office to schedule the initial consultation for the owner. Referrals should also be to a specific provider to remove any work on the owner's part to find a local veterinary nutritionist, behaviorist, and/or sports medicine and rehabilitation specialist. The veterinary team should also follow up with any referrals made to ensure the owner is in compliance with monthly follow-ups. Weight recheck appointments, whether at the primary or referral level, should be made in advance and confirmation reminders within 24 to 48 hours of the appointment are appropriate. Each recheck is an opportunity to document the pet's caloric intake and activity level, with comparisons made to previous data and the pet's current rate of weight loss. The SMART goals or implementation intentions should be reviewed and appropriate adjustments made based on the success or lack thereof.

Does the 5 A's System Work?

Implementation of the 5 A's system is not consistent in the human medical system, specifically as it pertains to obesity counseling at the primary care level. Barriers to success reported by physicians include not having enough time to discuss weight management during a routine primary care appointment[101,102] and a lack of readily available weight management educational materials.[103] A feeling of inadequate training to successfully discuss and treat obesity has been found on the part of the physician,[103–111] whereas others feel well prepared, but minimally effective.[102,112] From the patient perspective, assistance and arrangement are the constructs they most want their physicians to address, whereas advise and assess are actually most commonly used.[113] There is a similar pattern in the veterinary/animal obesity construct, with dog owners reporting weight discussions with their veterinarians, but disagreement with their veterinarian's assessment when their dog's BCS indicated an overweight status.[114] Underestimation of pet BCS has been noted with both cat[18,20,21,23,50] and dog[4,114–116] owners.

SUMMARY

Although the diet plays an integral part in weight management, environmental and behavioral treatment should be considered as part of a comprehensive weight loss plan for cats and dogs. Feeding strategies, exercise, and overall daily activity level are environmental aspects that need to be addressed. Specific behavior treatment strategies, geared toward both the pet and its owner, should also be addressed. In order to effectively adopt these strategies into clinical practice, the veterinary team should consider use of the 5 A's behavioral counseling approach. Although this approach will not guarantee success of the weight loss plan, it may help to improve overall owner adherence. It also provides the veterinary team with targeted strategies to recommend realistic plans and guides adjusting those plans throughout the weight loss phase.

REFERENCES

1. Krook L, Larsson S, Rooney JR. The interrelationship of diabetes mellitus, obesity, and pyometra in the dog. Am J Vet Res 1960;21:120–7.
2. Robertson ID. The association of exercise, diet and other factors with owner-perceived obesity in privately owned dogs from metropolitan Perth, WA. Prev Vet Med 2003;58(1–2):75–83.
3. McGreevy PD, Thomson PC, Pride C, et al. Prevalence of obesity in dogs examined by Australian veterinary practices and the risk factors involved. Vet Rec 2005;156(22):695–702.
4. Colliard L, Ancel J, Benet J-J, et al. Risk factors for obesity in dogs in France. J Nutr 2006;136(Suppl 7):1951S–4S.
5. Lund EM, Armstrong PJ, Kirk CA, et al. Prevalence and risk factors for obesity in adult dogs from private US veterinary practices. Int J Appl Res Vet Med 2006; 4(2):177–86.
6. Courcier EA, Thomson RM, Mellor DJ, et al. An epidemiological study of environmental factors associated with canine obesity. J Small Anim Pract 2010;51(7): 362–7.
7. Heuberger R, Wakshlag J. The relationship of feeding patterns and obesity in dogs. J Anim Physiol Anim Nutr (Berl) 2011;95(1):98–105.
8. Mao J, Xia Z, Chen J, et al. Prevalence and risk factors for canine obesity surveyed in veterinary practices in Beijing, China. Prev Vet Med 2013; 112(3–4):438–42.
9. Corbee RJ. Obesity in show dogs. J Anim Physiol Anim Nutr (Berl) 2012. http:// dx.doi.org/10.1111/j.1439-0396.2012.01336.x.

10. Lund EM, Armstrong PJ, Kirk CA, et al. Health status and population character-istics of dogs and cats examined at private veterinary practices in the United States. J Am Vet Med Assoc 1999;214(9):1336–41.

11. Edney AT, Smith PM. Study of obesity in dogs visiting veterinary practices in the United Kingdom. Vet Rec 1986;118(14):391–6.

12. Sallander M, Hagberg M, Hedhammar A, et al. Energy-intake and activity risk factors for owner-perceived obesity in a defined population of Swedish dogs. Prev Vet Med 2010;96(1–2):132–41.

13. Such ZR, German AJ. Best in show but not best shape: a photographic assess-ment of show dog body condition. Vet Rec 2015;177(5):125.

14. Scarlett JM, Donoghue S, Saidla J, et al. Overweight cats: prevalence and risk factors. Int J Obes Relat Metab Disord 1994;18(Suppl 1):S22–8.

15. Donoghue S, Scarlett JM. Diet and feline obesity. J Nutr 1998;128(Suppl 12): 2776S–8S.

16. Robertson ID. The influence of diet and other factors on owner-perceived obesity in privately owned cats from metropolitan Perth, Western Australia. Prev Vet Med 1999;40(2):75–85.

17. Russell K, Sabin R, Holt S, et al. Influence of feeding regimen on body condition in the cat. J Small Anim Pract 2000;41(1):12–7.

18. Allan FJ, Pfeiffer DU, Jones BR, et al. A cross-sectional study of risk factors for obesity in cats in New Zealand. Prev Vet Med 2000;46(3):183–96.

19. Lund EM, Armstrong PJ, Kirk CA, et al. Prevalence and risk factors for obesity in adult cats from private US veterinary practices. Int J Appl Res Vet Med 2005; 3(2):88–96.

20. Colliard L, Paragon B-M, Lemuet B, et al. Prevalence and risk factors of obesity in an urban population of healthy cats. J Feline Med Surg 2009;11(2):135–40.

21. Courcier EA, O'Higgins R, Mellor DJ, et al. Prevalence and risk factors for feline obesity in a first opinion practice in Glasgow, Scotland. J Feline Med Surg 2010; 12(10):746–53.

22. Courcier EA, Mellor DJ, Pendlebury E, et al. An investigation into the epidemi-ology of feline obesity in Great Britain: results of a cross-sectional study of 47 companion animal practises. Vet Rec 2012;171(22):560.

23. Cave NJ, Allan FJ, Schokkenbroek SL, et al. A cross-sectional study to compare changes in the prevalence and risk factors for feline obesity between 1993 and 2007 in New Zealand. Prev Vet Med 2012;107(1–2):121–33.

24. Corbee RJ. Obesity in show cats. J Anim Physiol Anim Nutr (Berl) 2014;98(6): 1075–80.

25. German AJ, Holden SL, Bissot T, et al. Dietary energy restriction and successful weight loss in obese client-owned dogs. J Vet Intern Med 2007;21(6):1174–80.

26. Bissot T, Servet E, Vidal S, et al. Novel dietary strategies can improve the outcome of weight loss programmes in obese client-owned cats. J Feline Med Surg 2010;12(2):104–12.

27. Wakshlag JJ, Struble AM, Warren BS, et al. Evaluation of dietary energy intake and physical activity in dogs undergoing a controlled weight-loss program. J Am Vet Med Assoc 2012;240(4):413–9.

28. Vitger AD, Stallknecht BM, Nielsen DH, et al. Integration of a physical training program in a weight loss plan for overweight pet dogs. J Am Vet Med Assoc 2016;248(2):174–82.

29. Gentry SJ. Results of the clinical use of a standardized weight-loss program in dogs and cats. J Am Anim Hosp Assoc 1993;29(4):369–75.

30. Laflamme DP, Kuhlman G, Lawler DF. Evaluation of weight loss protocols for dogs. J Am Anim Hosp Assoc 1997;33(3):253–9.

31. Michel KE, Bader A, Shofer FS, et al. Impact of time-limited feeding and dietary carbohydrate content on weight loss in group-housed cats. J Feline Med Surg 2005;7(6):349–55.

32. Brooks D, Churchill J, Fein K, et al. 2014 AAHA weight management guidelines for dogs and cats. J Am Anim Hosp Assoc 2014;50(1):1–11.

33. Saker KE, Remillard RL. Performance of a canine weight-loss program in clinical practice. Vet Ther 2005;6(4):291–302.

34. German AJ, Holden SL, Morris PJ, et al. Long-term follow-up after weight management in obese dogs: the role of diet in preventing regain. Vet J 2012;192(1): 65–70.

35. Laflamme D, Kuhlman G. The effect of weight-loss regimen on subsequent weight maintenance in dogs. Nutr Res 1995;15(7):1019–28.

36. Nagaoka D, Mitsuhashi Y, Angell R, et al. Re-induction of obese body weight occurs more rapidly and at lower caloric intake in beagles. J Anim Physiol Anim Nutr (Berl) 2010;94(3):287–92.

37. Deagle G, Holden SL, Biourge V, et al. Long-term follow-up after weight management in obese cats. J Nutr Sci 2014;3:e25.

38. Franz MJ, VanWormer JJ, Crain AL, et al. Weight-loss outcomes: a systematic review and meta-analysis of weight-loss clinical trials with a minimum 1-year follow-up. J Am Diet Assoc 2007;107(10):1755–67.

39. Anderson JW, Konz EC, Frederich RC, et al. Long-term weight-loss maintenance: a meta-analysis of US studies. Am J Clin Nutr 2001;74(5):579–84.

40. Diabetes Prevention Program Research Group, Knowler WC, Fowler SE, et al. 10-year follow-up of diabetes incidence and weight loss in the Diabetes Prevention Program Outcomes Study. Lancet 2009;374(9702):1677–86.

41. Anastasiou CA, Karfopoulou E, Yannakoulia M. Weight regaining: from statistics and behaviors to physiology and metabolism. Metabolism 2015;64(11): 1395–407.

42. Greenway FL. Physiological adaptations to weight loss and factors favouring weight regain. Int J Obes 2015;39(8):1188–96.

43. Clark M, Hampson SE, Avery L, et al. Effects of a tailored lifestyle self-management intervention in patients with type 2 diabetes. Br J Health Psychol 2004;9(Pt 3):365–79.

44. Bland I, Hill J. Tackling dog obesity by tackling owner attitudes. CAB review: perspectives in agriculture, veterinary science, nutrition and natural resources. CABI 2011;6(006):1–7.

45. Linder D, Mueller M. Pet obesity management: beyond nutrition. Vet Clin North Am Small Anim Pract 2014;44(4):789–806, vii.

46. Churchill J. Increase the success of weight loss programs by creating an environment for change. Compend Contin Educ Vet 2010;32(12):E1.

47. German AJ. Style over substance: what can parenting styles tell us about ownership styles and obesity in companion animals? Br J Nutr 2015;113(Suppl): S72–7.

48. Laflamme DP. Understanding and managing obesity in dogs and cats. Vet Clin North Am Small Anim Pract 2006;36(6):1283–95, vii.

49. Harper EJ, Stack DM, Watson TD, et al. Effects of feeding regimens on bodyweight, composition and condition score in cats following ovariohysterectomy. J Small Anim Pract 2001;42(9):433–8.

50. Kienzle E, Bergler R. Human-animal relationship of owners of normal and overweight cats. J Nutr 2006;136(Suppl 7):1947S–50S.

51. Bland IM, Guthrie-Jones A, Taylor RD, et al. Dog obesity: owner attitudes and behaviour. Prev Vet Med 2009;92(4):333–40.

52. Holmes KL, Morris PJ, Abdulla Z, et al. Risk factors associated with excess body weight in dogs in the UK (Abstract). J Anim Physiol Anim Nutr (Berl) 2007; 91(3–4):166–7.

53. Norris MP, Beaver BV. Application of behavior therapy techniques to the treatment of obesity in companion animals. J Am Vet Med Assoc 1993;202(5): 728–30.

54. German AJ, Holden SL, Mason SL, et al. Imprecision when using measuring cups to weigh out extruded dry kibbled food. J Anim Physiol Anim Nutr (Berl) 2011;95(3):368–73.

55. Burkholder WJ, Bauer JE. Foods and techniques for managing obesity in companion animals. J Am Vet Med Assoc 1998;212(5):658–62.

56. Levine ED, Erb HN, Schoenherr B, et al. Owner's perception of changes in behaviors associated with dieting in fat cats. J Vet Behav Clin Appl Res 2016;11: 37–41.

57. Kienzle E, Bergler R, Mandernach A. A comparison of the feeding behavior and the human-animal relationship in owners of normal and obese dogs. J Nutr 1998;128(Suppl 12):2779S–82S.

58. Murphy M, Lusby AL, Bartges JW, et al. Size of food bowl and scoop affects amount of food owners feed their dogs. J Anim Physiol Anim Nutr (Berl) 2012; 96(2):237–41.

59. Morrison R, Penpraze V, Beber A, et al. Associations between obesity and physical activity in dogs: a preliminary investigation. J Small Anim Pract 2013;54(11): 570–4.

60. Chan CB, Spierenburg M, Ihle SL, et al. Use of pedometers to measure physical activity in dogs. J Am Vet Med Assoc 2005;226(12):2010–5.

61. Warren BS, Wakshlag JJ, Maley M, et al. Use of pedometers to measure the relationship of dog walking to body condition score in obese and non-obese dogs. Br J Nutr 2011;106(Suppl 1):S85–9.

62. Chauvet A, Laclair J, Elliott DA, et al. Incorporation of exercise, using an underwater treadmill, and active client education into a weight management program for obese dogs. Can Vet J 2011;52(5):491–6.

63. Kushner RF, Blatner DJ, Jewell DE, et al. The PPET Study: people and pets exercising together. Obesity (Silver Spring) 2006;14(10):1762–70.

64. Morrison R, Reilly JJ, Penpraze V, et al. A 6-month observational study of changes in objectively measured physical activity during weight loss in dogs. J Small Anim Pract 2014;55(11):566–70.

65. Ellis SLH, Rodan I, Carney HC, et al. AAFP and ISFM feline environmental needs guidelines. J Feline Med Surg 2013;15(3):219–30.

66. Appelhans BM, French SA, Pagoto SL, et al. Managing temptation in obesity treatment: a neurobehavioral model of intervention strategies. Appetite 2016; 96:268–79.

67. Lowe MR, Butryn ML. Hedonic hunger: a new dimension of appetite? Physiol Behav 2007;91(4):432–9.

68. Desroches S, Lapointe A, Ratté S, et al. Interventions to enhance adherence to dietary advice for preventing and managing chronic diseases in adults. Cochrane Database Syst Rev 2013;(2):CD008722.

69. Webb TL. Why pet owners overfeed: a self-regulation perspective. Paper presented at the Companion Animal Nutrition Summit: the future of weight management. Barcelona (Spain): Nestle Purina; 2015. p. 89–94.
70. Cohen GL, Sherman DK. The psychology of change: self-affirmation and social psychological intervention. Annu Rev Psychol 2014;65:333–71.
71. Steele CM. The psychology of self-affirmation: sustaining the integrity of the self. Adv Exp Soc Psychol 1988;21:261–302.
72. Sherman DK. Self-affirmation: understanding the effects. Soc Personal Psychol Compass 2013;7(11):834–45.
73. Gollwitzer PM. Implementation intentions: strong effects of simple plans. Am Psychol 1999;54(7):493–503.
74. Gollwitzer PM. Goal achievement: the role of intentions. Eur Rev Soc Psychol 1993;4(1):141–85.
75. Koestner R, Lekes N, Powers TA, et al. Attaining personal goals: self-concordance plus implementation intentions equals success. J Pers Soc Psychol 2002;83(1):231–44.
76. Sheldon KM, Elliot AJ. Goal striving, need satisfaction, and longitudinal well-being: the self-concordance model. J Pers Soc Psychol 1999;76(3):482–97.
77. Sheldon KM, Houser-Marko L. Self-concordance, goal attainment, and the pursuit of happiness: can there be an upward spiral? J Pers Soc Psychol 2001;80(1):152–65.
78. Koestner R, Horberg EJ, Gaudreau P, et al. Bolstering implementation plans for the long haul: the benefits of simultaneously boosting self-concordance or self-efficacy. Pers Soc Psychol Bull 2006;32(11):1547–58.
79. Powers TA, Koestner R, Topciu RA. Implementation intentions, perfectionism, and goal progress: perhaps the road to hell is paved with good intentions. Pers Soc Psychol Bull 2005;31(7):902–12.
80. Webb TL, Sheeran P. Mechanisms of implementation intention effects: the role of goal intentions, self-efficacy, and accessibility of plan components. Br J Soc Psychol 2008;47(Pt 3):373–95.
81. Teixeira PJ, Carraça EV, Marques MM, et al. Successful behavior change in obesity interventions in adults: a systematic review of self-regulation mediators. BMC Med 2015;13:84.
82. Armitage CJ. A volitional help sheet to encourage smoking cessation: a randomized exploratory trial. Health Psychol 2008;27(5):557–66.
83. Armitage CJ, Norman P, Noor M, et al. Evidence that a very brief psychological intervention boosts weight loss in a weight loss program. Behav Ther 2014;45(5):700–7.
84. Grimshaw J, Eccles M, Tetroe J. Implementing clinical guidelines: current evidence and future implications. J Contin Educ Health Prof 2004;24(Suppl 1):S31–7.
85. Whitlock EP, Orleans CT, Pender N, et al. Evaluating primary care behavioral counseling interventions: an evidence-based approach. Am J Prev Med 2002;22(4):267–84.
86. Fitzpatrick SL, Wischenka D, Appelhans BM, et al. An evidence-based guide for obesity treatment in primary care. Am J Med 2016;129(1):115.e1–7.
87. Vallis M, Piccinini-Vallis H, Sharma AM, et al. Clinical review: modified 5 As: minimal intervention for obesity counseling in primary care. Can Fam Physician 2013;59(1):27–31.

88. Bland IM, Guthrie-Jones A, Taylor RD, et al. Dog obesity: veterinary practices' and owners' opinions on cause and management. Prev Vet Med 2010; 94(3–4):310–5.

89. Rowe E, Browne W, Casey R, et al. Risk factors identified for owner-reported feline obesity at around one year of age: dry diet and indoor lifestyle. Prev Vet Med 2015;121(3–4):273–81.

90. Nijland ML, Stam F, Seidell JC. Overweight in dogs, but not in cats, is related to overweight in their owners. Public Health Nutr 2010;13(1):102–6.

91. German AJ, Heath SE. Feline obesity: a medical disease with behavioral consequences. In: Rodan I, Heath S, editors. Feline behavioral health and welfare. 1st edition. St Louis (MO): Saunders; 2015. p. 148–61.

92. Kealy RD, Lawler DF, Ballam JM, et al. Effects of diet restriction on life span and age-related changes in dogs. J Am Vet Med Assoc 2002;220(9):1315–20.

93. Marshall WG, Hazewinkel HAW, Mullen D, et al. The effect of weight loss on lameness in obese dogs with osteoarthritis. Vet Res Commun 2010;34(3): 241–53.

94. Impellizeri JA, Tetrick MA, Muir P. Effect of weight reduction on clinical signs of lameness in dogs with hip osteoarthritis. J Am Vet Med Assoc 2000;216(7): 1089–91.

95. Mlacnik E, Bockstahler BA, Müller M, et al. Effects of caloric restriction and a moderate or intense physiotherapy program for treatment of lameness in overweight dogs with osteoarthritis. J Am Vet Med Assoc 2006;229(11):1756–60.

96. Hoenig M, Thomaseth K, Waldron M, et al. Insulin sensitivity, fat distribution, and adipocytokine response to different diets in lean and obese cats before and after weight loss. Am J Physiol Regul Integr Comp Physiol 2007;292(1): R227–34.

97. Biourge V, Nelson RW, Feldman EC, et al. Effect of weight gain and subsequent weight loss on glucose tolerance and insulin response in healthy cats. J Vet Intern Med 1997;11(2):86–91.

98. Yaissle JE, Holloway C, Buffington CAT. Evaluation of owner education as a component of obesity treatment programs for dogs. J Am Vet Med Assoc 2004;224(12):1932–5.

99. German AJ, Holden SL, Gernon LJ, et al. Do feeding practices of obese dogs, before weight loss, affect the success of weight management? Br J Nutr 2011; 106(Suppl 1):S97–100.

100. Doran GT. There's a S.M.A.R.T. way to write management's goals and objectives. Manage Rev 1981;70(11):35–6.

101. Ruelaz AR, Diefenbach P, Simon B, et al. Perceived barriers to weight management in primary care–perspectives of patients and providers. J Gen Intern Med 2007;22(4):518–22.

102. Al-Ghawi A, Uauy R. Study of the knowledge, attitudes and practices of physicians towards obesity management in primary health care in Bahrain. Public Health Nutr 2009;12(10):1791–8.

103. Forman-Hoffman V, Little A, Wahls T. Barriers to obesity management: a pilot study of primary care clinicians. BMC Fam Pract 2006;7:35.

104. Alexander SC, Ostbye T, Pollak KI, et al. Physicians' beliefs about discussing obesity: results from focus groups. Am J Health Promot 2007;21(6):498–500.

105. Fogelman Y, Vinker S, Lachter J, et al. Managing obesity: a survey of attitudes and practices among Israeli primary care physicians. Int J Obes Relat Metab Disord 2002;26(10):1393–7.

106. Ferrante JM, Piasecki AK, Ohman-Strickland PA, et al. Family physicians' practices and attitudes regarding care of extremely obese patients. Obesity (Silver Spring) 2009;17(9):1710–6.
107. Jelalian E, Boergers J, Alday CS, et al. Survey of physician attitudes and practices related to pediatric obesity. Clin Pediatr (Phila) 2003;42(3):235–45.
108. Salinas GD, Glauser TA, Williamson JC, et al. Primary care physician attitudes and practice patterns in the management of obese adults: results from a national survey. Postgrad Med 2011;123(5):214–9.
109. Bocquier A, Verger P, Basdevant A, et al. Overweight and obesity: knowledge, attitudes, and practices of general practitioners in france. Obes Res 2005;13(4):787–95.
110. Kristeller JL, Hoerr RA. Physician attitudes toward managing obesity: differences among six specialty groups. Prev Med 1997;26(4):542–9.
111. Jochemsen-van der Leeuw HGA, van Dijk N, Wieringa-de Waard M. Attitudes towards obesity treatment in GP training practices: a focus group study. Fam Pract 2011;28(4):422–9.
112. Campbell K, Engel H, Timperio A, et al. Obesity management: Australian general practitioners' attitudes and practices. Obes Res 2000;8(6):459–66.
113. Sherson EA, Yakes Jimenez E, Katalanos N. A review of the use of the 5 A's model for weight loss counselling: differences between physician practice and patient demand. Fam Pract 2014;31(4):389–98.
114. White GA, Hobson-West P, Cobb K, et al. Canine obesity: is there a difference between veterinarian and owner perception? J Small Anim Pract 2011;52(12):622–6.
115. Courcier EA, Mellor DJ, Thomson RM, et al. A cross sectional study of the prevalence and risk factors for owner misperception of canine body shape in first opinion practice in Glasgow. Prev Vet Med 2011;102(1):66–74.
116. Eastland-Jones RC, German AJ, Holden SL, et al. Owner misperception of canine body condition persists despite use of a body condition score chart. J Nutr Sci 2014;3:e45.

Communicating with Pet Owners About Obesity

Roles of the Veterinary Health Care Team

Julie Churchill, DVM, PhD[a],*, Ernie Ward, DVM, CVFT[b]

KEYWORDS

- Obesity • Weight management • Client communication • Transtheoretical model
- Stages of change • Veterinary health care team roles • Human animal bond

KEY POINTS

- Treating pet obesity continues to challenge veterinary health care professionals.
- Elements of a successful weight loss program include client commitment, an individualized treatment plan integrating the needs the needs of the client, pet, and their environment, and a reassessment plan.
- Training and enlisting all members of the veterinary care team will improve the effectiveness of addressing pet obesity.
- Communication tools can be used to assess the client's ability to change and implement a weight loss plan at the right time in the right way to achieve better adherence and improve patient health.

INTRODUCTION

Obesity continues to be the most prevalent disease of dogs and cats, affecting up to half of the nation's pets.[1–5] Although it is well established that obesity negatively influences health, well-being, and even lifespan,[3–6] veterinary professionals continue to struggle to educate and convince clients to begin or adhere to a weight loss program for their pets. Veterinarians may lack the leadership, communication training, or educational tools to effectively implement the team skills and protocols within their clinics[7,8] to improve the standard of care of patients. This often creates a cultural identity crisis within the veterinary health care team and deployment of inconsistent medical and communication standards. In addition, lack of time, apprehensions about poor revenue, and concern over inadequate treatments are additional barriers to talking about pet

Dr J. Churchill serves on the Nestle Purina Advisory Council. Dr E. Ward has nothing to disclose.
[a] Department of Veterinary Clinical Sciences, University of Minnesota College of Veterinary Medicine, C-339, 1352 Boyd Avenue, Saint Paul, MN 55108, USA; [b] Association for Pet Obesity Prevention, E3 Management, LLC, Ocean Isle Beach, NC 28469, USA
* Corresponding author.
E-mail address: churc002@umn.edu

obesity with clients. Veterinary teams must present a consistent and unified group approach to effectively address pet obesity and overcome these challenges.

Many veterinarians are reluctant to tell a pet owner their animal is obese.[9] Veterinarians fear this information will offend, upset, anger, or even lose a client. This imagined outcome leads to professional anxiety, apprehension, and avoidance.[10] Veterinary team members prefer to ignore issues that make them uncomfortable. When veterinarians offer dietary recommendations, their medical advice is often disregarded or a patient fails to achieve the desired weight loss, leading to further discourage veterinary teams from confronting nutritional issues. Small animal obesity is a complex, challenging, and sensitive topic. It is a professional responsibility to address pet obesity as any other serious disease. Effective communication and treatment strategies must be designed to involve the staff and actively engage clients to successfully combat the pet obesity epidemic.

TEAM APPROACH TO NUTRITIONAL COUNSELING

Consistency is necessary for sustainable success in any endeavor. Veterinary teams need a clear, logical, and methodical approach to consistently and effectively counsel clients on a pet's diet, lifestyle, and quality of life. Nutritional counseling and weight loss recommendations should be integrated into routine vaccination visits, during puppy and kitten appointments, and during sick pet visits. Every veterinary team's goal should be to assess a patient's nutrition as the fifth vital sign in every examination, as proposed by the World Small Animal Veterinary Association.[11] Although the specific workflow and techniques may vary between clinics and practitioners, it is essential each veterinary team has an organized system or protocol for acquiring and delivering medical advice to clients. The nutritional counseling workflow should be based on a team's nutritional competency and dietary philosophy, individualized communication styles of team members and clientele, and infrastructure constraints, such as number of staff, examination rooms, length of appointments, and equipment.

Another important element to ensure nutritional counseling is successful is to assure that the health care team is open-minded, approachable, and empathetic. Many pet owners are reluctant to ask a veterinary health care professional for dietary advice. They may feel embarrassed, concerned their choices will be judged or labeled as a "bad pet parent," or they are unconvinced the veterinary team can help them. Clients may also view veterinary clinics as limited in resources or knowledge and only offer advice on the few products they sell. These concerns are legitimate doubts that the veterinary profession must address. Veterinary teams must be proactive on weight loss and nutritional counseling; clients may rarely broach the subject unprompted. Each team member must be trained to consistently communicate in a nonthreatening, nonjudgmental, and caring manner. Veterinarians must focus on actively listening to clients, being open-minded and flexible to individual pet owner's needs, and offering individualized support. Every team member has the opportunity to influence a pet owner's understanding of body condition, nutrition, and commitment to change. It is the responsibility of veterinarians and team leaders to create and maintain best practices for communications and treatments. Nutritional counseling is now a minimum standard of veterinary care and should be included in every patient interaction.

THE 3 ELEMENTS FOR WEIGHT LOSS SUCCESS

Clinical success in achieving and maintaining weight loss in pets is determined by 3 key factors: (1) owner commitment, (2) individualized weight loss program, (3) regular and consistent veterinary contact. When all 3 elements are simultaneously combined, success rates are greatly improved.[12]

Owner Commitment

Psychologists have established numerous models to help explain how and why humans make changes in behavior to improve health. The "stages of change" model developed by Prochaska and colleagues,[13] also known as the transtheoretical model, can be used to assess a person's readiness to change his or her behavior.[14] Prochaska's model can help veterinary professionals better understand the change process, successfully partner with pet owners, and customize recommendations that best suit each client's needs—in other words, to use the right approach for the right client at the right time. Implementing a weight loss plan when the client is ready to act on this advice will improve success and more efficiently use the veterinary team's time and resources.

Identify the pet owner's stage of change

The transtheoretical model identifies 5 stages of change and their characteristic attributes.[12–14]

1. *Precontemplation*. The person has no intention of taking action in the next 6 months. These clients might commonly be referred to as resistant, unmotivated, or unaware, but clearly, they are not ready or willing to change. In reality, pet obesity intervention programs are often inappropriate and ineffective for these individuals.
2. *Contemplation*. The person is aware of the pros and cons of changing a particular habit or lifestyle action and intends to change in the next 6 months. These clients may be stuck "thinking about it," intending to change "soon."
3. *Preparation (decision making)*. The person plans to take action in the next month or sooner. Clients may have recognized the problem of their pet's weight and already sought advice from books, online sources, or a pet store employee, trainer, or veterinary professional.
4. *Action*. The person has taken action that is significant enough to reduce the risks for disease. For example, the client may have reduced the number of treats fed or selected a different pet food. However, a change is not considered a significant action unless it has reduced calories by at least 10% and provided complete and balanced nutrition.
5. *Maintenance*. The person continues action to prevent relapse.

Select a stage-appropriate intervention

Many weight loss programs fail because the type of intervention chosen is not accurately matched to the client's readiness to change (**Table 1**).[12] Many traditional pet obesity programs are action-oriented, but most clients do not start in the action stage. By understanding the stages of change, veterinary health professionals can adapt their communication strategies to better meet a client's stage of readiness and support the client to become ready for change. It may take time and several visits to establish rapport and build the trust necessary to move clients along to the next stage. These visits may require patience and understanding, but the patient's health needs can be better served and great loyalty can be built when partnered with these clients.

1. *Precontemplation*. If a client is in this stage, it is not yet time to try implementing a weight loss plan for the pet. However, it is equally important not to ignore the patient's obesity until the next annual examination. A frequent monitoring plan should be implemented for these patients. Express concern about the pet's health and recommend monthly follow-ups to monitor for any adverse effects of

Table 1
Assessing readiness for change

Stages of Change	Common Client Comments at This Stage	Strategies for the Health Care Team	Communication Options for Veterinary Health Care Team
Precontemplation: Lack of awareness of the problem or does not intend to make changes at the present	"Tigger is supposed to be big! You know he's part Maine coon." "Mocha's big boned; her father weighed 160 lbs of solid muscle!" "I think she's cute this way, not all skin and bones." "Buddy's always begging and my husband gives him all those treats."	Seek permission to talk more about the problem. Provide general information. Establish a supportive relationship and express concerns. Leave the door open for future discussion.	"Do you have time to talk about Tigger's weight today?" "It's easy to see how much you love Tigger and want the best for him." "I am concerned that Mocha's weight may be contributing to her health problems. What do you think?" "It seems like you are comfortable with her weight right now; yet I'm a little worried about how it can impact her health later." "What are your thoughts about Buddy's weight?"
Contemplation: Aware there is a problem, but is not yet necessarily ready to change their behavior. This is often where people become "stuck" and need to learn more about the issues involved	"Yes, but...." "I might be able to fit another walk into my busy day." "We could try reducing the amount of table scraps. He has come to expect a treat every time he goes potty."	Look at pros/cons of change and identify supports and barriers. Talk about ambivalence. Empathize with client's difficulties surrounding change.	"It seems like you are concerned about Tigger's weight but it may not be the right time for a weight management plan with all you have going on in your life." "What is the most important part of your relationship with Buddy?" "What will be most difficult for you?" "What changes seem like they will be easiest piece to put into place?" "What time of day does he beg the least?" "Who in your family can help you with Mocha?" "I know it's hard to do this when you are already busy."

Stage	Example client comments	Provider role	Example provider statements
Decision making (preparation): A commitment to change is made, and plans are set to do the best they can	"What can I do to address Tigger's weight?" "What was the name of that weight-reducing diet we might try?" "I know it's harmful to be this heavy." "We're ready to do this!"	Help determine the best course of action and aid in setting small, specific, achievable goals. Partner with client to create an individualized plan.	"What are your goals concerning Tigger's weight?" "What small change might you make to start with?" "How might we work together to develop a weight loss plan for Tigger?" "I hear you saying that you would like to discuss a plan to address Tigger's weight." "What part of your feeding program would you really hate to change?" "You seem ready to address Buddy's weight." "I'm confident she will feel better."
Action: The client is ready and is making changes	"I am walking her twice a day now." "She seems to like the weight-reduction diet and eats it readily."	Provide active support, encouragement, and praise client's efforts. Celebrate success and share their enthusiasm.	"It sounds like you are doing a great job of increasing Buddy's activity." "What changes have you noticed in Mocha?" "It sounds like your plan is working well for you and Tigger."
Maintenance: The client is progressing with the changes	"I am starting to look forward to the monthly weigh-ins, as I am anxious to see how much she has lost."	Provide active support to maintain and practice new behaviors. Praise client's efforts and recognize progress. Celebrate success and empathize with challenges. Plan for minor setbacks.	"Due to your hard work, she lost one pound in the past month. We can see the difference in her." "What has been the most challenging for both of you?" "What's worked the best for these challenges?" "Can I share some other ideas?" "Everyone is so pleased with the progress you are making with Tigger's weight." "Winter can be hard when you can't get outside as often. Let's plan some strategies."
Lapses: The client lapses into old habits	"We did not make any progress in Buddy's weight this month. My kids came home and everyone gave him treats." "We were doing well until I had the baby. I just don't have any time for Mocha these days."	Identify changes that have worked and use these as strategies for moving forward. Understand that motivation comes and goes as a normal part of life. Plan ahead for lapses.	"It's hard to be consistent with any health plan. At times we will do better than others." "What has been working well for you and Mocha?" "How might we capitalize on these successes?" "How do you feel we should proceed from here?"

Client comments can give an indication of their stage of change as well as help the health care team identify strategies and communication options to better match their readiness for change.

being overweight. Depending on the patient's health, these can be brief weight checks performed by a technician. Conveying care and concern for the patient rather than judgment allows the team to follow both the patient and the client while being prepared to initiate a weight loss treatment plan when the client is more receptive.

2. *Contemplation.* If a client seems to be "stuck" in this stage, he or she may need to learn more about the issues involved. Providing resources such as handouts or links to reliable Web sites may give them necessary information and reinforce the message that you care about their pet's health and that obesity is a real health concern.

3. *Preparation.* Recruit these clients for action-oriented programs. Ask them what they need to be ready to begin and how the veterinary team can help them.

4. *Action.* Work with clients to design an individual weight loss plan that accounts for their pet's needs and their own schedule and lifestyle. Provide feedback and compliments on the patient's progress to encourage the client to stay with the plan.

5. *Maintenance.* Refine the plan as necessary to achieve or continue healthy weight loss. Giving clients information and permission for a possible relapse removes judgment if a relapse should happen and encourages them to seek your help if it does. Talk with them about potential challenges they anticipate in the future and proactively strategize some possible solutions.

Individualized Weight Loss Plan

Every pet patient is unique and requires an individualized weight loss plan for optimal success. Partner with the client to create a customized plan that works for the family and meets the nutritional requirements of the pet. A careful and complete diet history (eg, food and treat types, amounts, schedule)[15] can reveal important information about how the family relates to the pet through food and often provides insight about potential challenges for the client. Examples of diet history forms have been published previously[15,16] and provide useful tools that can also reveal information about the pet's nutritional status, which is often imbalanced from excess treats and human foods being added to the commercial pet food. Because pets' energy needs can vary significantly, it is important to know an individual pet's current caloric intake. The diet history can help provide this information, which can then serve as a much more accurate starting point for calculating the pet's specific food dose (for initial weight loss, start at 75% to 80% of current caloric intake[4,17]). (See Deborah E. Linder and Valerie J. Parker's article, "Dietary Aspects of Weight Management in Cats and Dogs," in this issue, for more detail on determining appropriate caloric intake for a weight loss plan.)

Reassess the Patient's Progress

Initially, biweekly follow-up visits help to support clients, ensure a healthy rate of loss (0.5% to 2%[4] body weight/week), and detect potential relapses or challenges early so that the weight loss plan can be adjusted or the client can be redirected before additional weight gain occurs and frustration becomes another barrier to success.

ENLIST THE VETERINARY HEALTH CARE TEAM TO IMPLEMENT NUTRITIONAL RECOMMENDATIONS

Perhaps the most important decision a pet owner makes each day regarding their pet's health is what they feed it. In most cases, diet selection, feeding frequency and amounts, and treating habits are established without veterinary consultation.

The veterinary profession must aggressively take steps to reclaim nutritional expertise with pet owners. The most effective method is to incorporate nutrition into every appointment.

TYPICAL VETERINARY WEIGHT LOSS VISIT WORKFLOW

1. *Previsit (Client).* Before each annual or wellness appointment, e-mail a brief client and patient health and diet questionnaire. Inform the client that taking the time to complete the short checklist will expedite their appointment and allow the veterinarian to focus on their chief concerns. Use open-ended questions such as, "Describe your typical day's feeding and treats." Include additional information, such as activities, number of other pets, indoor and outdoor time, parasite prevention, sleep habits, and other medical or behavioral concerns. Ask the client to take a picture of their pet food label, a typical feeding amount, and food and water bowls. If the client is unable to e-mail or message the pictures, tell them you can view them together during the appointment.Regardless of whether the client completes these forms, you have the opportunity to subtly emphasize topics such as nutrition, behavior, and parasite prevention. Before their visit, a staff member reviews the questionnaire and calculates approximate daily caloric intake and the percentage of calories from treats.
2. *Clinic Check-In (Front Staff and Technician).* Staff member verifies client contact information, reviews or collects diet and medical history information. The pet is weighed and an initial Body Condition Score[16] (BCS) is obtained. This check-in is an excellent time to take pictures of the pet to document current weight status and BCS. Veterinary team members have tremendous opportunity to positively influence a client's attitude toward obesity and diet while obtaining the medical history and check-in. Communicate in a confident and encouraging manner, avoid derogatory or apologetic terms, and focus on solutions.
3. *Examination (Veterinarian and Technician).* The technician reviews pertinent medical history and vital sign data with the veterinarian and with the client. The veterinarian performs a physical examination and nutritional assessment and constructs treatment plans based on findings and client concerns. Additional diagnostic tests may be recommended based on the patient's needs. A typical weight loss plan includes the following:
   - Specific food and treat recommendations
   - Daily feeding amounts and treat allocation
   - Frequency or feeding management (ie, food puzzles, environmental enrichment and activity or exercise plans)
   - Monitoring plan (ie, monthly weight checks, repeat BCS, morphometrics)
4. *Postexamination Review (Technician).* The technician reviews the veterinarian's written examination report and treatment plan. It is critical that the staff member is trained to address the client's doubts during this stage. Many clients will use this opportunity in the absence of the attending veterinarian to reveal their true anxieties or fears about implementing change. Share personal testimonies and success stories and offer support during the weight loss process to allay fears. If the client is disinterested, remain positive and allow future opportunities for change. Review therapeutic diets or recommend foods, provide pet food measuring foods cups, encourage food puzzles, and review feeding instructions. Schedule a telephone call-back in 3 to 5 days.
5. *Discharge and Check-Out (Front Staff).* Verify the client has possession of all items dispensed and understands instructions. Review treatment plan goals and

objectives and schedule recheck visits. Provide positive reinforcement and encouragement. "You're going to be thrilled when you see how much better Rover feels after getting in shape!"

6. *Recheck and Reweigh Visits (Technician and Veterinarian).* E-mail a previsit brief questionnaire asking how the pet is responding to the diet or lifestyle change, any treatment challenges, and questions for the veterinary team. Pictures or videos of any concerns or issues are welcome. At the time of the appointment, the veterinary staff weighs the pet, obtains a BCS and any additional morphometrics, and calculates the rate of weight loss. The veterinarian determines if any changes to the weight loss program are necessary. A written recheck examination report with subsequent clinical steps is provided to the client.

TEAM TRAINING

A team approach to pet weight loss should be centered around a shared belief that nutrition is the "best medicine." Every member of the health care team should have a clearly defined role and understand their importance in providing the best health care for their patients. Successful veterinary clinics conduct regular staff training or medical rounds to practice how to deliver consistent communication in the most effective manner. Mutual support and teamwork are only accomplished through consistent practice and training. Team members recognize that good listening abilities may be the most important component of effective client communication and use active listening skills. Every staff member, including front desk, assistants, and auxiliary help, should be trained to answer basic questions regarding the clinic's nutritional philosophy and key points about any specific diets you recommend.

Other attributes of successful pet weight loss programs include

- Successful teams "walk the talk" when it comes to veterinary nutrition. Evaluate and assess staff members' personal pet's feeding habits and dispel any myths the team may have about veterinary nutrition, weight loss, and exercise programs. Providing personalized veterinary nutritional counseling for all staff members is an excellent way to teach nutrition in a relatable, nonthreatening, and meaningful manner and demonstrate convincing results.
- Create a cohort of veterinarians and technicians in your practice to be in-clinic champions for nutrition and weight loss. Provide these team members with additional training opportunities and rewards for accomplishments (job titles, public recognition, pay incentives).
- Develop and implement written protocols that clearly define the roles and responsibilities of every member of the health care team to ensure that every patient has a nutritional assessment and receives a dietary recommendation at every visit.
- Use a routine medical record review process to ensure the clinic's nutritional protocols are being executed.
- Staff members share personal experiences with the clinic's recommended diets, weight loss products, feeding management ideas, exercises, and other proposals with clients.

TEAM COMMUNICATION SKILLS

Collaborative communication or relationship-centered care[18] must be presented by the entire veterinary team. This communication technique encourages veterinary clients to become more actively involved in their pet's care. Relationship-centered care also uses shared decision making between the client and veterinary team. This technique uses a "together we can" approach instead of the traditional "the veterinarian tells you to" tactic.

The first step toward a team relationship–centered weight loss plan is recognition of an existing or emerging excess weight problem. This recognition can be accomplished by simply creating a protocol that requires veterinary staff to review and document the pet's last recorded weight and BCS. Most dogs and cats are examined annually[19] in the United States, making year-to-year weight and BCS comparisons easily accessible. Consistently evaluating each patient's previous body weight and BCS is the foundation for a successful weight loss program. Teaching pet owners to perform body condition scoring is another important measure in weight management and can be verified and reinforced at each visit.

The next step is to determine a pet owner's feeding habits. It is important for veterinary team members to use inviting open-ended questions such as, "Tell me how you feed your dog throughout the day," or "What does a typical day's feeding and treating look like at the Smith household?," instead of more clinical, closed-ended questions such as, "What brand of food do you feed?" or "How much do you feed your cat?" Open-ended questions are more likely to reveal important details and initiate a conversation about a pet owner's feeding habits and dietary beliefs than narrowly defined, closed-ended inquiries. Instead of asking, "Do you give Buddy treats or table scraps?," try saying, "Tell me about Buddy's favorite human foods or snacks." This type of question implies the team understands and accepts the importance of treats in the client's relationship with their pet. The best predictors of acceptance and adherence to a weight loss program are the veterinary professional's interviewing skills and the qualities of the veterinary–client interaction.[20] The conversations the veterinary team initiates concerning diet, lifestyle, and attitudes help build trust and establish a client's interest and willingness in a weight loss program or nutritional counseling. It is critical to provide adequate staff training and allow ample time with clients to increase success.

It is important the veterinary staff avoids using words such as "fat," "heavy," "chubby," "plump," or other derogatory terms. It is also essential that staff members do not passively diminish the importance of obesity by making statements such as, "He's not that fat. I've seen worse," or "Most pets need to lose a little weight." Minimizing the potential severity of excess body fat undermines future attempts at weight loss counseling. The goal at this point in the communication process is to gather information, not make a diagnosis or pronounce judgment. Veterinarians should strive to create a clinic culture that understands and values preventive care, especially diet, lifestyle, and body condition and seeks ways to enhance compassionate communication to support medical recommendations.

If weight gain or excess weight is identified, the staff needs to alert the veterinarian by directly reviewing the patient's medical history with the attending veterinarian, sharing medical notes, or other means of transferring clinical information. When dealing with an overweight or obese veterinary patient, it is imperative the veterinarian remain calm, convey compassion and concern, and emphasize the importance of achieving and maintaining a healthy weight.

VETERINARY COMMUNICATION

Talking about nutrition and excess weight with pet owners can be problematic without prior thought and training. Few subjects are as emotionally loaded and full of personal opinions as what and how people feed their pets. Veterinarians may worry they will inadvertently offend a client, are not comfortable with their nutritional knowledge, or think they are too busy to engage in a "food debate." All of these factors have contributed to the pet obesity epidemic.

Despite the challenges associated with addressing pet obesity, ignorance and evasion is infinitely worse. The best communication practices begin with honesty; if a pet is overweight, tell the owner. Avoid the derogatory terms and focus on the pet's quality of life. The battle against obesity is not about chasing a number on a scale; it is about improving health and decreasing disease. Guide the conversation toward daily activities such as feeding and treating habits, walks and play activities, climbing stairs, and getting in and out of cars. Inquire about inappropriate elimination in cats, the inability to jump onto beds or chairs, or withdrawal from contact and interaction. Focus on the relationship between pet and pet owner and how better veterinary nutrition can improve quality of life and prevent debilitating and expensive diseases such as type 2 diabetes, osteoarthritis, hypertension, cancer, and more.

COMMUNICATION CHALLENGES: OBESE CLIENTS

Many veterinarians avoid discussing a pet's obesity with an overweight or obese client because they fear they may inadvertently offend the client. Although this can certainly occur, it is rare. The risks of offending a client can be minimized by adopting a nonthreatening communication approach when discussing pet obesity.

Begin with an open body posture. Ideally, the veterinary team member will be seated and positioned at a 45° angle to the client without any table or other barrier between the care provider and the client. Most American and western European clients are most comfortable talking to a medical professional at a 2- to 3-foot distance from their closest body part.[21–23] Avoid crossing legs or arms and holding a medical record or having a computer between the veterinarian and the client. Maintain good eye contact and speak in a normal, warm tone. Remember that this conversation is about the pet's health, not the client's weight issues. Assume the client may know that their pet is overweight but does not understand the negative health effects of obesity. If the health care team member preloads their thoughts with ideas about the client's weight, then nonverbal communication will convey their discomfort and nervousness. If a client perceives the veterinarian is uncomfortable or unconfident, they will disregard their advice.

Open the pet obesity conversation with a statement acknowledging the relationship between the pet and owner:

Mrs. Guild, I know how much you care for Skippy and that's why I want to discuss his weight. As a veterinarian, it's my job to keep updated on advances in medicine and how to keep Skippy as healthy and happy as possible. Numerous studies conclude if a pet is overweight their risk of developing diabetes, arthritis, high blood pressure, and even many types of cancer is increased. What do you think about Skippy's current weight?

I suppose he's a little heavy like the rest of us.

You're right. Skippy's not alone in his battle against obesity. Veterinarians are often trained to focus on getting our patients to a certain weight, no matter what. I think we should take a slightly different approach with Skippy. I want us to focus our efforts on improving Skippy's overall health and well-being so that he can be around for a long time. How does that sound?

Oh anything I can do to help Skippy. He's my baby.

By directing the conversation away from a specific weight and number and toward quality of life and health, the discussion can be subtly shifted toward the health of the pet with little risk of offending anyone, regardless of how sensitive they may be. Then the discussion of diet, exercise, goals, and quality of life can begin in a more collaborative setting. Avoid approaching the issue directly and saying, "Skippy's getting a little full around the middle. His ideal weight should be about 10 pounds less. We need to get him on a diet to get those pounds off." This tactic will likely be met with defensiveness and reluctance to follow the recommendations.

COMMUNICATION CHALLENGES: OBESE VETERINARIANS

Overweight or obese veterinarians may be disinclined to discuss weight loss with their clients because they may be uncomfortable with their own body condition. If a veterinarian is struggling with their own weight and diet, be honest and proactive. By stating the obvious, discussing personal weight loss challenges, an overweight veterinarian can transform a potentially anxious exchange into a calm and meaningful conversation. Of course, a veterinarian using this approach must be sincerely seeking help and actively pursuing lifestyle and dietary changes.

> *Mrs. Howe, I'd like to take a few minutes to discuss Rover's weight gain. I know how much he means to your family and that you want him to be as healthy and lively for as long as possible. As you can plainly see, I'm like the majority of Americans who share Rover's weight problem and the potential medical problems that accompany obesity. And, like Rover, I want to be around a long time and see my kids grow up and kiss my future grandkids. In order for me to do that and to be able to do things I want to do with them, I'm working on getting fit. As you probably know, this is not easy for pets or people, but I'd like to share with you some strategies that I have found successful for both my own pets and my patients.*

By reframing the discussion in personal terms and immediately transferring the focus to the pet's condition, you will be seen as truthful, caring, and concerned, attributes every veterinarian should strive for with any client interaction and which ultimately lead to increased adherence to our recommendations, regardless of the topic.

COMMUNICATING WITH A DISINTERESTED CLIENT

Not every client is ready to discuss their pet's weight. Although we do not want to force the issue or appear overzealous, the problem still needs to be addressed and for future revisitation.

> *As we've mentioned, I'm concerned about Freddie's weight gain.*

> *Yeah, well he's a house cat and he's going to be fat.*

> *You're absolutely right. Indoor cats have a higher incidence of weight problems and the associated diseases such as diabetes than outdoor cats. The great news is if Freddie sheds as few as 2 or 3 pounds, it can reduce his risk of those diseases. I'm also glad Freddie lives inside your safe home; I don't advocate cats living outdoors in our area—it's simply too dangerous. I'm going to send you home with some information on food choices for indoor cats that I'd like you to look over when you have some time. You may be surprised at how easy some of the steps we can take to help our pets lose weight and live healthier. Since he's gained more weight over this past year, I think we should follow-up in 3 months instead of waiting a year before we see him again.*

Make this point politely, review the major health risks associated with being overweight, and keep the emphasis on health and quality of life. The key is to continue discussing obesity in the face of adversity and not shut down or dismiss the client as "difficult." Many clients will eventually take action, and if the veterinary team has remained helpful, positive, and proactive, the client will return. If the pet owner feels vilified, judged, or uncomfortable, they will likely seek help from a pet store or other nonprofessional.

SUMMARY

Nutritional counseling is now a minimum standard of veterinary care and should be included in every patient interaction. The veterinary team has a professional obligation to address pet obesity as any other serious disease. In order to successfully combat the pet obesity epidemic, the entire health care team must be involved and armed with effective communication and treatment strategies to actively engage clients. It is the responsibility of veterinarians and team leaders to create and maintain best practices for communications and treatments. Every team member has the opportunity to influence a pet owner's understanding of a healthy body condition, nutrition, and commitment to change. Clinical outcome can be greatly improved by assessing the client's readiness for change so team members can enlist different communication tools and timing of when to implement obesity treatment plans, tailored to the individual pet. Successfully managing obesity can be very rewarding. The pet achieves an improved quality of life and greater health, and the pet owner becomes a loyal client when he or she is an active partner in the health care plan.

REFERENCES

1. Association for Pet Obesity Prevention. Available at: www.PetObesityPrevention.org. Accessed January 27, 2016.
2. Lund EM, Armstrong PJ, Kirk CA, et al. Prevalence and risk factors for obesity in adult cats from private US veterinary practices. Intern J Appl Res Vet Med 2005; 3(2):88–96.
3. Obesity: epidemiology, pathophysiology and management of the obese dog. In: Pibot P, Biourge V, Elliot D, editors. Encyclopedia of canine clinical nutrition. Aimargues (France): Royal Canin; 2006. p. 11–6.
4. Brooks D, Churchill J, Fein K, et al, American Animal Hospital Association. 2014 AAHA weight management guidelines for dogs and cats. J Am Anim Hosp Assoc 2014;50(1):1–11.
5. Colliard L, Paragon BM, Lemuet B, et al. Prevalence and risk factors of obesity in an urban population of healthy cats. J Feline Med Surg 2009;11(2):135–40.
6. Kealy RD, Lawler DF, Ballam JM, et al. Effect of diet restriction on life span and age related changes in dogs. J Am Vet Med Assoc 2002;220:1315–20.
7. National Research Council. Workforce needs in veterinary medicine. Washington, DC: The National Academies Press; 2013. p. 99–101.
8. Coates C. Veterinary practice management. 1st edition. Wallingford, Oxfordshire (United Kingdom): Centre for Agriculture and Biosciences International; 2013. p. 63–6.
9. Trone Brand Energy/Association for Pet obesity prevention proprietary research. Reprinted by permission. 2014.
10. Strategies to Overcome and Prevent Obesity Alliance. Why weight? A guide to discussing obesity and health with your patients. Available at: http://www.stop obesityalliance.org/wp-content/themes/stopobesityalliance/pdfs/STOP-Provider-Discussion-Tool.pdf. Accessed January 27, 2016.

11. World Small Animal Veterinary Association. Nutritional assessment guidelines. 2011. Available at: http://www.petnutritionalliance.org/pdfs/pna-nutritional assessment.pdf. Accessed January 27, 2016.

12. Churchill J. Increase the success of weight loss programs by creating an environment for change. Compend Contin Educ Vet 2010;32(12):E1.

13. Prochaska JO, Johnson S, Lee P. The transtheoretical model of behavior change. In: Shumaker SA, Ockene JK, Riekert KA, editors. The handbook of health behavior change. 3rd edition. New York: Springer; 2009. p. 59–84.

14. Buffington CA, Holloway C, Abood SK. Contemporary issues in clinical nutrition. In: Buffington CA, Holloway C, Abood SK, editors. Manual of veterinary dietetics. St Louis (MO): Saunders; 2004. p. 143–62.

15. Michel KE. Using a diet history to improve adherence to dietary recommendations. Compend Contin Educ Vet 2009;31:22–4.

16. Baldwin K, Bartges J, Buffington T, et al. AAHA nutritional assessment guidelines for dogs and cats. J Am Anim Hosp Assoc 2010;46(4):285–96.

17. Perea S. Treating an overweight patient with hip pain. Clin Brief 2010;8:63–5.

18. Cornell KK, Kopcha M. Client-veterinarian communication: skills for client centered dialogue and shared decision making. Vet Clin North Am Small Anim Pract 2007;37:37–47.

19. American Veterinary Medical Association. U.S. pet ownership and demographics sourcebook (2012). Schaumburg (IL): American Veterinary Medical Association; 2012.

20. Morrisey JK, Voiland B. Difficult interactions with veterinary clients: working in the challenge zone. Vet Clin North Am Small Anim Pract 2007;37:65–77.

21. The Health Care Communication Group. Writing, speaking, and communication skills for health professionals. New Haven (CT): Yale University Press; 2001. p. 249–79.

22. Rankin HJ. Power talk: the art of effective communication. Step Wise Press; 1999.

23. Pease A, Pease B. The definitive book of Body Language. New York City: Bantam Books; 2006.

Obesity Prevention and Weight Maintenance After Loss

Alexander James German, PhD[a,b]

KEYWORDS

- Dog • Cat • Overweight • Nutrition • Regain • Prophylaxis

KEY POINTS

- The process of inappropriate weight gain is insidious and many animals are at risk.
- Treatment of obesity is challenging and affected animals frequently fail.
- To prevent obesity, veterinary professionals should establish a program of body weight monitoring and body condition scoring assessments, starting during growth and then continuing throughout adult life.
- Body weight should be monitored regularly during the phase after weight loss to identify animals at risk of rebound.
- Feeding a therapeutic weight management diet during the weight maintenance phase significantly decreases the risk of regain.

INAPPROPRIATE WEIGHT GAIN IN DOGS AND CATS
Definition

Inappropriate weight gain typically arises from persistent dietary caloric intake in excess of maintenance requirements, leading to increased adipose tissue deposition. It is a major and ever increasing concern in companion animals and, depending on the degree increased adiposity, is classified as either overweight or obese. A dog or cat whose weight exceeds 10% of its optimal is classified as being overweight, and the term obese is used to define animals whose weight is 20% greater than optimal.[1]

The author has nothing to disclose.
The author's academic post is funded by Royal Canin. The author has also received financial remuneration and gifts from a number of companies (including Royal Canin, WALTHAM, Hill's Pet Nutrition, Nestle Purina, and Zoetis) for providing educational material, speaking at conferences, and consultancy work. Research funding has also been obtained from various commercial companies including Royal Canin, WALTHAM, and Zoetis.
[a] Institute of Ageing & Chronic Disease, University of Liverpool, Leahurst Campus, Chester High Road, Neston CH64 7TE, Merseyside, UK; [b] Institute of Veterinary Sciences, University of Liverpool, Leahurst Campus, Chester High Road, Neston CH64 7TE, Merseyside, UK
E-mail address: ajgerman@liverpool.ac.uk

Prevalence of Inappropriate Weight Gain

There have been various peer-reviewed studies determining the prevalence of obesity and overweight, which suggest that 29% to 39% and 19% to 29% of dogs and cats, respectively, may be affected.[1] Most concerning is that the problem is becoming increasingly more prevalent, with a recent survey suggesting that the affected population of dogs and cats has increased by 37% and 90%, respectively, in the last 5 years.[2] Further, companion animal obesity is now of global significance, with a recent survey demonstrating that 44% of dogs in China were now classified as overweight.[3]

Onset of Inappropriate Weight Gain

A recent cohort study demonstrated that, for cats that become overweight later in life, body weight gradually increases through their adult years.[4] This is consistent with findings of cross-sectional epidemiologic studies that demonstrate that, in both dogs and cats, the relative prevalence of overweight is relatively low early in life, peaks during the middle-aged years, and lessens again later in life,[5,6] most likely as a result of the development of chronic diseases of old age. Thus, rather than developing suddenly, inappropriate weight gain is a gradual process that begins during early adult life, with adipose tissue accumulating gradually throughout the middle age years. This insidious pattern of onset can prove challenging both for owners and veterinarians because it is easily missed. Proactive monitoring is essential to spot the problem early and enable corrective measures to be implemented (see below).

Risk Factors for Inappropriate Weight Gain

A number of risk factors are known to predispose to the development of obesity in dogs and cats,[1,5,6] as outlined below.

Coexisting health problems
Many other diseases can alter energy flux, either by increasing energy intake or decreasing expenditure, and these can predispose to inappropriate weight gain (**Box 1**).

Rapid early life weight gain
In humans, a fast rate of growth predicts the likelihood of being obese during adulthood.[7] A similar phenomenon has also been reported in cats,[4] with genetic factors thought to be responsible.[8] However, it is not yet known whether rapid growth rates are a similar risk factor in dogs.

Box 1
Diseases that might predispose to inappropriate weight gain by altering energy flux

- Hyperadrenocorticism causes polyphagia and can predispose to increased energy intake.
- Side effects of some drugs, for example, glucocorticoids and anticonvulsants include polyphagia, which again might lead to weight gain.
- Neutering is a risk factor for inappropriate weight gain (see below), and may be required for treatment of diseases like pyometra.
- Orthopedic diseases decreases energy expenditure by decreasing physical activity.
- Hypothyroidism decreases energy expenditure by decreasing basal metabolic rate.

Breed

The prevalence of obesity is greater in certain dog breeds (eg, Labrador Retrievers, Golden Retrievers, Pugs, Cocker Spaniels, Beagles, and mixed breed dogs), but less in other breeds.[6] This suggests that, as in humans,[9] genetic influences are an important risk factor. In cats, associations have not been demonstrated consistently between the development of obesity and pedigree cat breeds. Instead, mixed breed cats (especially the domestic shorthair) are at greatest risk. Nonetheless, genetic factors are suspected to be responsible for the rapid early life weight gain, which is itself a risk factor for obesity in adult life.[8]

Age

As discussed, the peak prevalence of overweight cats and dogs is during the middle-aged years (6–19 years in dogs and 5–11 years in cats).[5,6] Prevalence is less, but not zero, during the growth phase and during the senior years, the latter probably because of the development of chronic diseases that lead to body weight loss.

Sex and neutering

Male cats were predisposed to obesity in 1 study[10]; in contrast, female dogs are more likely than male dogs to be overweight.[6,11] In both species, neutering is an important risk factor, most likely because the alterations in sex hormones lead to changed behavior, most specifically increased food seeking and decreased physical activity.[12,13]

Behavioral factors

Abnormal feeding behaviors have also been implicated as possible risk factor for the development of feline obesity,[14] for example, the cat being more anxious or not properly controlling its food intake.

Environment and activity

Both cats and dogs that live indoors, especially in apartments, are more likely to be overweight than those who go outdoors.[15–17] In addition, those cats living either with dogs or with 1 to 2 other cats are also predisposed to becoming obese.[15,16]

Dietary factors

The role that diet plays in the development of obesity has not yet been clarified, because variable results have been seen in different studies. A summary of key findings from the studies conducted are reported in **Box 2**.

Owner factors

A number of owner factors have also been implicated in the development of obesity in dogs and cats (**Box 3**).

OUTCOMES OF WEIGHT MANAGEMENT

Various studies have examined the outcomes of weight loss programs in both obese pet dogs and cats.[24–26] Most commonly, only short-term assessments are considered (eg, 2–6 months only), and only simple outcomes reported (eg, initial rate of weight loss and overall percentage weight loss). These results give the mistaken impression that weight loss programs are highly successful in both species. Studies examining rates and percentage weight loss over the whole of a weight loss cycle (eg, long enough to return the animal to their ideal weight) are more representative,[27,28] but still do not give a complete picture of overall success. In 1 study that examined a weight loss intervention that included client education, only 53% of dogs completed the 6-month trial period.[25] A completion rate of 60% was reported for an entire weight

---

Box 2
Dietary factors associated with overweight or obesity in dogs and cats

- No association between diet type and obesity in cats.[15,18]
- Dry food as risk factor for development obesity in young cats.[17]
- Dietary fat content, rather than carbohydrate associated with obesity in cats.[19]
- Feeding free choice seems to increase the risk of obesity in cats.[15,16]
- An association between numbers of meals and snacks and obesity in dogs.[20]
- Feeding of table scraps associated with obesity in cats and dogs.[15,16,20,21]
- Cat or dog present when food is prepared.[15,16,20,21]
- 'Grocery store' dog foods positively associated with canine obesity.[18]
- 'Premium' cat foods positively associated with feline obesity.[5]

---

loss cycle (eg, start to reaching target weight) in a more recent study,[29] with various reasons cited for noncompletion including development of other diseases, poor compliance with the program, and personal reasons of the owner (eg, owner illness, bereavement in the family). The main factors associated with failure to comply were the degree of obesity (more obese dogs are less likely to complete a program) and slower rates of weight loss.

These findings are consistent with other research that has highlighted that weight loss becomes increasingly challenging the longer an animal is on their weight loss program.[30,31] In the early stages of weight loss (eg, first 2–3 months), both dogs and cats can be expected to lose at approximately 1% body weight per week, which is what most clinicians would recommend as safe weight loss. Thereafter, the rate of weight loss begins to slow down and, to maintain rates of weight loss, dietary energy intake must be reduced, usually by 10% to 20% during the course of a period of weight loss.[30,31] However, rate of weight loss declines despite this such that, after 12 months of a program, rates of weight loss are usually less than 0.3% per week in both dogs and cats. Such slowing of progress can be frustrating to owners and, perhaps, explains why compliance, which is good in the first 2 to 3 months (typically >80% in both species), worsens gradually as time goes on.[30,31]

Box 3
Owners factors implicated in the development of overweight and obesity in dogs

- Lower average income for owners of overweight dogs,[18,22] but not cats.[23]
- Overhumanization of the dog by the owner is associated with obesity in dogs.[18]
- Cat used by owner as a human companion substitute.[23]
- Close observation of feeding behavior of the cat or dog.[18,23]
- Less time spent playing with cat.[23]
- Owner obesity positively associated with obesity in dogs[18] and cats.[23]
- Owners of obese cats less interested in preventive health[18,23]
- A stronger owner–animal bond is reported between obese cats and their owners.[14]

Furthermore, success should not simply be viewed in terms of what happens during the weight loss period. Arguably, it is more important to ensure that any weight lost is not regained. Indeed, this is a common problem with human diet-based weight loss programs, where the majority of subjects regain weight, and some regain more than they originally lost.[32] Recent studies have demonstrated that regain is also a problem in obese companion animals, with 48% of dogs and 46% of cats rebounding.[33,34] In dogs, the magnitude of rebound is typically less severe than in humans, with approximately 10% of dogs regaining more than 50% of the weight they originally lost. Cats are intermediate, with approximately one-third regaining more than 50% of the weight they had lost. These findings highlight the fact that weight management should never be considered simply in terms of the weight loss phase. Because long-term success involves many of the risk factors that contributed to the initial inappropriate weight gain remain after the program is completed, and veterinary professionals must therefore focus as much effort into prevention of rebound as for the preceding weight loss phase (see below).

The results summarized in this section clearly highlight that long-term success is relatively disappointing when it comes not only to reaching target weight successfully, but also maintaining that loss. If approximately one-half of dogs and cats that start a weight loss plan reach target, and only one-half of those maintain their weight loss subsequently, only a minority (approximately one-quarter) derive long-term benefit. However, there is a further factor that must be considered when looking at success of weight management therapy, namely, what proportion of obese animals actually undergo weight loss in the first place. To the author's knowledge no study has as of yet addressed this issue. That said, recent studies have highlighted that veterinarians discuss weight status and body condition with owners of overweight dogs in less than 2% of all consultations.[35,36] This suggests that only a minority of overweight animals are identified and the issue discussed with their owner. The number that actually start a weight loss plan is likely to be substantially less than this.

Few obese dogs and cats start a weight loss program, and only a minority of those that do successfully lose weight and keep it off subsequently. This suggests that therapy for obesity is far from perfect. As a consequence, a new approach is needed to manage this epidemic, instead focusing on prevention rather than cure.

TOOLS FOR OBESITY PREVENTION

As discussed, the challenges faced with successfully losing weight after and keeping it off mean that it makes more sense to prevent inappropriate weight gain from developing in the first place. This can be more challenging than it sounds, not least because the problem develops insidiously, such that it is often missed until it is too late. Prevention of obesity is a lifelong problem, requiring interventions right from the early growth phase through to the senior adult years. It requires the veterinary professional to pay constant attention to maintaining a neutral energy balance (in terms of dietary energy intake relative to energy expenditure) while at the same time confirming this through regular monitoring of body weight and condition. Although the main tools for obesity prevention are similar, the strategy adopted is different at different stages, which are considered separately.

Monitoring Strategies

Body weight
Arguably, taking regular bodyweight measurements is the most important monitoring strategy for preventing inappropriate weight gain and, provided that the same set of

calibrated electronic scales is used, it is much more precise and objective than other approaches (eg, body condition scoring [BCS], using a tape measure). Even small deviations from optimal weight can be spotted quickly enabling early intervention. Items such as clothing or harnesses should be removed, if possible, and the animal should be positioned so that they are standing with all 4 feet on the scales. The animal should also be as still as possible during the weighing process, and the result should be recorded immediately in the animal's case notes (to 2 decimal places for all cats and small breed dogs, and 1 decimal place for medium to giant breed dogs). If not doing so already, veterinary clinics should instigate a policy of weighing all animals at every single visit because, over time, an individualized historical record of body weight will be available for all registered patients.

Body condition

BCS is the most widely accepted clinical method of assessing body composition because it is very quick and easy to perform, while at the same time being reliable. It is important that the veterinary professional conduct the assessment, because owners underestimate the condition of their pet. Various BCS systems have been described, but the World Small Animal Veterinary Association Global Nutrition Committee recently made a recommendation that the 9-point system be universally adopted.[37] As well as determining current weight status (underweight, optimal weight, overweight), knowledge of the current BCS can be used to estimate optimal weight, should it deviate from normal (**Box 4**).

Other methods for determining body condition

In addition to regular assessments of body weight and periodic BCS, other methods can also be considered including zoometry, bioimpedance, and advanced body composition assessments. Zoometry involves measuring bodily dimensions with a tape measure, and can either be single measurements to informally assess aspects of overall shape (eg, body circumference measurements) or multiple measurements that are combined in a formal zoometric system.[38,39] However, although such systems do correlate with body fat mass, there can be variability in measurements taken with a tape measure,[40] and the systems are more cumbersome to use taking longer than assessing BCS. Bioimpedance techniques for assessing body fat mass have also been described, and handheld machines are available. However, the lack of reliability

---

Box 4
Estimating ideal bodyweight from current bodyweight and body condition score

It is estimated that each unit between 5 and 9 on the 9-point body condition system approximates to 10% of additional bodyweight. After weighing the animal, and assessing body condition scoring (BCS), a simple calculation can then be used to estimate the ideal weight:

Ideal weight = Current weight × (100 ÷ [100 + 10 × {current BCS − 5}])

Example

For an animal weighing 40.0 kg with a current body condition score of 8 of 9 (ie, about 30% overweight), the ideal weight can be calculated as follows:

40 kg × (100 ÷ [100 + 10 × {8−5}]) = 30.8 kg

Always be aware that such calculations only ever provide an estimate of ideal weight, and can be prone either to overestimation or underestimation of actual ideal weight. It is advisable for the veterinary professional to monitor body condition during the weight loss process, and make adjustments if needed.

means that results can be misleading.[41] Finally, advanced measures have been described for assessing body composition more accurately in small animals, including dual-energy x-ray absorptiometry and computed tomography.[42,43] These techniques have limited application for primary care practice, and are more suited to a referral setting, should the need arise.

Determining Metabolizable Energy Requirements and Energy Expenditure

To help with proactive monitoring, knowledge of an animal's metabolizable energy requirements for maintenance (MER) at different life stages is useful, and predictive equations for different stages of life have been reviewed and reported.[44,45] However, although such equations are accurate on average, the specific requirements for an individual can deviate markedly. Therefore, after calculating expected MER with such an equation, the exact requirements should be adjusted on a trial an error basis, for example, by taking serial measurements of bodyweight, and adjusting food intake accordingly (see below).

Research methodology is available for measuring energy expenditure (a proxy measure for MER), with techniques including indirect calorimetry and tracer studies involving, for example, doubly labelled water.[46] Indirect calorimetry has been adopted as a clinical measure in humans,[47] and portable indirect calorimeters have been developed. The clinical use of indirect calorimetry has also been validated for dogs.[48] However, this technique has not yet found a wide clinical application in the veterinary field.

Dietary Strategies

To best frame discussions regarding diet and food intake, a nutritional assessment is recommended, ideally in accordance with the recent recommendations of the World Small Animal Veterinary Association Global Nutrition Panel.[37] Such an assessment will enable the individual needs of the animal to be taken into account when setting the prevention strategy to adopt. Dietary strategies that can help in preventing inappropriate weight gain include determining the most appropriate main meal to feed, adopting a responsible plan for providing treats and extra food, accurate measurement of food portions, managing feeding activity within and outside the home, and adapting food intake as nutritional requirements change.

Periodically, it is advisable to reappraise the animal's nutrition (again using the World Small Animal Veterinary Association Nutritional assessment), because actual feeding regimens can 'drift' gradually over time. Such a review helps to refocus priorities, adjust the strategy if there have been changes in circumstance, and ensure continued commitment from the owner in preventing weight gain.

Main meal feeding

All dogs and cats should be fed a diet that is nutritionally complete and balanced and, preferably, tailored to the correct life stage, be it for growth, the early adult period, or for the senior years. If the current diet is appropriate, and both owner and pet are happy with it, then there is no need to change. Instead, attention should be focused on ensuring that the correct amount is being fed for requirements, and adjusted as needs change. Particular care should be focused when changing to a new diet (**Box 5**).

For dogs and cats that show marked food seeking behavior or excessive begging, a change of food type can be considered. The same characteristics as those used in a purpose-formulated weight loss food will also help for weight maintenance. For example, food can be supplemented with protein and fiber, and these formulations are known to minimize signs of hunger and reduce voluntary food intake in both dogs and cats.[24] Increasing food volume can also reduce voluntary food intake, for

---

Box 5
Advice on procedures for introducing a new food, and adjusting intake to ensure energy intake remains in balance

- Introduce it gradually, over 5 to 7 days, to avoid any gastrointestinal disturbances.
- Calculate the correct amount of food to feed, based on the animal's maintenance energy requirements, if known. If not known, follow the manufacturer's guidelines, adjusted to the animal's individual circumstances, for example, its current body weight, breed, sex, neuter status, activity level, and so on.
- Feed the food for a 2-week period and reweigh the animal. If the weight has remained stable, continue to feed the same amount of food; if the bodyweight has decreased, increase the amount fed by 5% to 20% (depending on the amount of weight lost), and reweigh after another 2 weeks; if the bodyweight has increased, decrease the amount fed by 5% to 20% (depending on the amount of weight gained), and reweigh after another 2 weeks.

Once bodyweight is known to be stable, continue to weigh the animal at regular intervals to ensure that weight remains on track.

---

instance, by adding water (or using a wet food) or expanding a kibbled food with air. Finally, the shape of a kibbled diet can also be altered, which can force a dog or cat to chew food more, thereby slowing intake.

Accurate portion size measurement
In addition to accurately determining MER, it is critical that there is both precision and accuracy when measuring food portions. This is most important for dry food because it is so energy dense, and small errors can lead to large differences in actual energy intake. Although measuring cups may be the simplest method of measuring dry food, they are unreliable, and can lead to overfeeding especially for small portion sizes (such as those fed to small dogs and cats).[49] For those animals known to be at risk of inappropriate weight gain or overeating, more accurate measurements are critical, and a different method is strongly recommended, if possible, using digital gram scales. In practice, it takes very little additional time in measurement and gives owner and veterinary professional reassurance that correct portions are being delivered day in and day out. Other methods that are currently in development include 'smart bowls' and computer-controlled food hoppers, which include gram scales within them, and automatically measure out the correct portion with the minimum of effort.

Responsible feeding of treats and extra food
It is critical to control the feeding of extra food, such as tidbits, table scraps, treats, and food scavenging. Most owners frequently are not aware of the contribution that such food sources can make to the daily ration. During the initial nutrition review, time should be taken to obtain a detailed understanding of the extra food the animal receives, and, to make this as accurate as possible, it is advisable to question multiple family members. In theory, it is preferable to avoid feeding any additional food, because there is a danger that it may make an otherwise balanced main meal unbalanced. In reality, most owners will not accept this because rewarding their pet is such an instinctive behavior. The solution is to develop a formal program of treating, which either makes use of existing food or, instead, permits the owner to use a controlled number of approved treats, to a maximum of 10% of MER, so as to ensure that the diet remains in balance overall. The energy content of such treats should be calculated and the amount of main meal fed should be reduced accordingly.

Ideally, human food and table scraps should still not be fed. To minimize temptation, it is best to ensure that pets are not in the kitchen area where food is being prepared and not allowed access to the dining area during meal times. Food preparation areas and dinner tables should be cleared before the pets are allowed back in, and trash bins and food stores should be properly secured. Finally, care should be taken when dogs are taken for walks. If scavenging at this time is a problem, it may be necessary for the dog to wear a muzzle or not be let off the lead.

Methods of feeding

Again, the initial nutritional assessment should include a discussion of how the owner feeds their pet(s). Most commonly, dogs will be given 1 to 2 main meals each day, and meal feeding in also common for cats, although some owners will leave food out all day. The latter should be discouraged, not least in multiple animal environments and with cats that are unable to regulate their daily food intake (see below).

It is worth considering the use of puzzle feeders as part of the overall feeding strategy. These are an excellent method of slowing food intake, thereby extending the feeding period. Not only does it help to minimize overeating (because there is more time for gastrointestinal hormones that lead to satiation to be released and affect the hunger center in the brain), but it also is more enjoyable for the pet.

In multiple pet households, it is critical to ensure that each has their own tailored feeding plan and only receives its own food. Various strategies can be used (**Box 6**). It can be a particular challenge when managing multiple cat households with 1 grazer cat (that is in ideal weight) and an overweight cat that does not regulate intake. Food should never just be left out and, instead, pets in the same household must be fed separately. For example, a grazer that can self-regulate can be allowed long periods to be fed, whereas the cat that tends to overeat is given food by puzzle feeder. Alternatively, food could be left out for the grazer in a location that the overweight cat cannot access (on a high surface, within a small 'creep' area—eg, box or cupboard with small hole through which the overweight cannot pass), using a smart bowl to allow free access for the grazer, while meal feeding or using a puzzle feeder in the overweight cat.

If desired, food can be given in 2 or more meals per day, preferably providing more food at times when the owner is with the pet (because this is when begging is most likely to occur). However, use of an interactive feeding device is preferred (eg, puzzle feeding toy or modified feeding bowl). These devices have the effect of slowing food intake, thereby improving satiety.

Physical Activity

In addition to controlling food intake, promoting energy expenditure is a valuable means of helping to prevent inappropriate weight gain. The main approach in both

---

Box 6
Strategies for ensuring separate feeding of individuals for multi-animal households

- Meal feeding animals in separate locations.
- Feeding in the same location but supervising food intake and picking food up when animals have finished.
- Using individual smart bowls programmed to recognize the microchip of the animal.
- Using separate feeding strategies for different pets (eg, meal feeding one, and using a puzzle feeder for another; meal feeding a cat that cannot regulate while providing a separate location or smart bowl for a cat that is a grazer).

cats and dogs is to increase physical activity, which has a modest but significant effect on energy expenditure in most animals. Indeed, in a recent canine study, each 1000 steps of walking increased energy expenditure by 1 kcal per kg 0.75 of body weight.[50] In addition to burning calories, physical activity can improve and maintain cardiovascular and musculoskeletal fitness, and improve the owner–pet bond. Regular daily sessions are recommended for both species, although the approach varies (**Table 1**). For dogs, at least 1 daily walk of 30 minutes is recommended. When play sessions are used in cats, short periods are sufficient activity, typically 1 to 2 minutes at a time 2 or more times per day.

The recommended exercise should take account of any concurrent medical concerns, and also be tailored to the capabilities of the pet. For example, if a dog has an orthopedic disease (such as osteoarthritis), controlled forms or exercise, such as leash walking are preferable to vigorous activity (off-leash running and playing with a ball). Alternatively, hydrotherapy could be used, depending on the cost and availability in the local region. Finally, the agreed plan should also take account on the preferences and capabilities of the owner, in terms of the time available, timing, and type of exercise.

A final method that can help to promote movement in both cats and dogs is the use of puzzle feeders, hollow toys in which you place a small amount of kibbled food. The cat or dog must then play with the toy to remove the food. Most animals rapidly learn how to use these, and will play for extended periods, often well after the toy is empty.

RECOMMENDATIONS FOR MONITORING STRATEGIES
Early Life Prevention

The importance of ensuring that dogs and cats grow at an appropriate rate during their early years cannot be overemphasized because this is the foundation to a healthy weight for the whole of the adult years. Epidemiologic studies in humans have demonstrated that inappropriate growth is a predictor of obesity later in life.[7] Indeed, a rapid rate of growth, catch-up growth (where an underweight for age child grows faster than average), and high early life body mass index are all independently associated with the risk of obesity at 7 years of age. A recent study has also demonstrated rapid growth to be a risk factor for later-life obesity in cats.[4] To the author's knowledge, no similar studies have as of yet been done in dogs. However, given that this effect seems to be conserved across 2 species, an important effect of growth on the risk of inappropriate weight gain in the future is likely also to exist in dogs.

Given such an importance to the growth period, regular monitoring of body weight throughout the growth phase is essential. Indeed, growth standards are now widely used in human pediatrics, with the most commonly adopted being those endorsed by the World Health Organization. Such growth standards enable appropriately trained health workers to monitor individual growth in children and verify that it is appropriate compared with a healthy reference population.[51] Regular weight monitoring can then

Table 1 Methods of promoting physical activity in dogs and cats	
Dog	**Cat**
Walking (on or off leash)	Play activity using fish rod toys
Play activity using balls, Frisbees, etc	Motorized toys
Hydrotherapy	Puzzle feeders
Puzzle feeders	Climbing frames and activity centers
Free exercise outdoors (in yard or garden)	Allow outdoor access (eg, cat flap)

be performed, and guidance can be given should the child's growth deviate from optimal. Unfortunately, such growth standards are not yet available for cats and dogs, and this can make charting healthy growth more challenging. Nonetheless, the principles of regular growth monitoring can still be applied to both dogs and cats. Recommendations for weight monitoring during growth are shown in **Box 7**.

Monitoring Strategy for Adult Animals

Inappropriate weight gain is an insidious phenomenon, and the early adult years are a particular period of risk. Indeed, the prevalence of overweight animals steadily increases in this period to a peak in mid adult life. Therefore, regular and proactive monitoring is critical as a means of identifying at risk animals, and making early corrections to prevent animals becoming overweight. The main recommendations for prevention of inappropriate weight gain during adult life are shown in **Box 8**.

Monitoring Strategy for the Postneutering Period

Neutering is a risk factor for inappropriate weight gain in both dogs and cats, although its influence varies among individuals. As a consequence, close monitoring of body weight and condition is essential during the postneutering period (**Box 9**).

Monitoring Strategy for Senior Animals

Weight checks should be continued into the senior life stage. Not uncommonly, activity can decline at this stage, not least because of concurrent diseases such as osteoarthritis have developed. Any increases in weight should prompt a nutritional and lifestyle review, with adjustments made as required. Of course, old age is also a time when chronic diseases are common, many of which can lead to loss of body weight, and especially body mass. Thus, the clinician should be alert to this possibility, and any unexpected decline in body weight should be investigated proactively to elucidate the cause. It is also common for animals to gain adipose tissue while at the same time losing

---

Box 7
Recommendations for weight monitoring during growth in cats and dogs

- Weight should first be recorded at first vaccination and recorded again at second vaccination. At this stage, the importance of healthy weight and healthy growth should be discussed with the owner, and a growth monitoring plan be implemented. Nutrition for growth can also be discussed.

- Body condition scoring should also be performed regularly during this time. Although systems have not been validated fully in growing animals, they can still provide guidance as to whether the weight is appropriate for the age.

- Ideally, regular weight and condition score checks should be performed on a monthly basis until the animal has reached its mature body weight (approximately 12 months for cats, 12–24 months for dogs). Compliance can be improved if these checks are coordinated with other preventive medicine visits for example, worming, neutering and microchipping, and so on.

- If weight gain is deemed to have occurred too rapidly or too slowly, adjustments to the nutrition plan can be made, which should have the effect of slowing subsequent growth to get the animal back on track.

- Pay particular attention to any animal that grows rapidly because this is likely to put them at increased risk of being overweight later in life. Owners should be forewarned that a rigorous policy of weight monitoring will also be essential for the adult years.

- Careful monitoring of the postneutering period to prevent weight gain associated with the postneutering period (see **Box 8**).

Box 8
Recommendations for prevention of inappropriate weight gain in adult cats and dogs

- Be aware of the risk factors for inappropriate weight gain (see Risk factors for inappropriate weight gain). Monitor at-risk animals closely throughout their adult years. Be especially alert to cats that gain weight rapidly during the growth phase; these cats are likely to be unable to regulate their food intake. Avoid free access to food (especially a dry kibbled diet), and accurately measure food portions so as to prevent overeating.

- Perform a number of weight measurements around the time of physical maturity and combine these with assessment of body condition scoring (BCS). Provided that the animal is in optimal condition (BCS 4–5/9) when this 'early adult weight' is recorded, the weight can then be used as the healthy weight for the whole of the adult years.

- Once the individual healthy adult weight is known, implement regular weight checks throughout the adult years to ensure that weight remains stable. It is preferable to use changes in body weight to determine the need for adjustments, rather than using BCS. This is because body weight measurements are more objective, easier to perform, and can identify much smaller changes than can BCS. In this respect, body weight changes of 0.5% can readily be identified using properly calibrated electronic scales. In contrast, a change in body weight of approximately 10% is typically required before the BCS changes by 1 BCS unit (on the 9-integer scale).

- Alterations to feeding and lifestyle should be considered if a change in bodyweight is identified between veterinary visits. Of course, it is up to the attending veterinary professional to determine whether or not intervention is necessary, and the exact intervention required. The author's recommended intervention points are as follows:
  - Greater than 2% change in body weight over a period of 7 days
  - Greater than 5% change in body weight over a period of 4 weeks
  - Greater than 10% change in body weight over a period of 6 months.

- Be aware if there are any changes to the animal's routine, for example, change of diet, change in activity pattern, or development of a concurrent disease. Consider more regular monitoring of body weight during these times, and make adjustments to the nutritional plan as required.

- As for growing animals, monitor the postneutering period carefully, so as to avoid inappropriate weight gain at this stage (see **Box 9**).

- Consider implementing different feeding methods (eg, puzzle feeders, smart bowls) if the owner is finding it challenging to limit food intake.

---

muscle mass. For this reason, regular assessment of body condition is also vital, and this should include a subjective assessment of muscle condition.[37] For most senior animals, checks every 6 months are sufficient. However, more regular monitoring should be considered for animals known to have a chronic disease that causes loss of body weight for example, chronic kidney disease and hyperthyroidism.

Prevention of Rebound After Weight Loss

As mentioned, subsequent regain of body weight is a common occurrence after successful weight loss in obese dogs and cats, with about one-half of those reaching target weight that are affected.[33,34] In dogs, the main factor that decreases the odds of such a rebound occurring is the food that is fed during the weight maintenance phase.[33] In this respect, weight regain is far less likely in those that continue to be fed the same purpose-formulated food that was used during the weight loss phase, than for dogs whose diets are switched to a different diet (eg, a standard canine maintenance diet or 'light' maintenance diet). In cats, the main factor associated with weight regain is age, with cats less than 9 years of age being at greater risk than cats greater

---

Box 9
Recommendations for monitoring for inappropriate weight gain in the postneutering period

- Measure body weight and body condition scoring (BCS) at the time of neutering to ensure that the dog or cat is in optimal condition.
- Reweigh 2 weeks after neutering, for example, at the time of suture removal.
- Reweigh at 4 weeks after neutering.
- If neutered as an adult, reweigh at 12 weeks, and then every 6 months thereafter. If body weight increases by greater than 5%, then make adjustments to the nutritional plan (eg, decrease food intake by 10%) then reassess weight every 2 weeks, making further adjustments until weight is stable again.
- If neutered during the growth phase, reweigh according to the usual practice policy, for example, on a monthly basis. Consider plotting weight change on a graph because this will enabled a 'neutering bounce' (more rapid and inappropriate gain of weight after neutering) to be identified more readily. If seen, make adjustments to the nutritional plan (eg, decrease food intake by 10%) then reassess weight 2 weeks later, making further adjustments until rate of growth is back on track.

---

than 9 years of age.[34] Therefore, particularly close monitoring of the period after weight loss is essential for younger cats. As for dogs, the author recommends that these cats continue with the purpose-formulated diet that was used during weight loss. The reason why older cats are less at risk of regain is not known, but may be related to the onset of chronic diseases during the senior years, many of which can leading to insidious weight loss. Therefore, there is less of a need to remain on the purpose-formulated weight loss diet (as for a young cat or dog) and, instead, a food should be selected that is appropriate to the life stage and or concurrent disease. Nonetheless, regular monitoring of body weight and body condition should continue, with adjustments being made to ensure weight is stable. The author's recommended plan for proactive monitoring of the weight maintenance phase is shown in **Box 10**.

Box 10
Recommendations for preventing regain of body weight after successful weight loss in an obese dog or cat

- Once target weight is reached, increase food intake by a small increment (eg, 5%–10%) and reweigh the animal 2 weeks later.
- If there has been further weight loss at the next revisit, increase by a further 5% to 10% and reweigh after a further 2 weeks.
- If weight regain has occurred at the next revisit, decrease food intake by one-half the amount of the last increment (eg, decrease by 5% if you increased by 10% initially), and reweigh after a further 2 weeks.
- Repeat the process of adjustments (eg, further small increments or decreases and weight checks every 2 weeks) until weight is stable between checks.
- Once weight is stable after 2 weeks, continue to reweigh, but gradually extending the interval for example, every 4 weeks, every 8 weeks, and then every 3 months. Thereafter, weight checks should be continued on a regular basis. For most animals, this can be according to the usual practice protocol for adult animals at the appropriate life stage. However, for animals at particular risk of regain (eg, those that lost more weight during their weight loss period, young cats, cats known to be unable to regulate their food intake), more regular checks could be considered.

SUMMARY

The process of inappropriate weight gain is insidious, and many animals are at risk of becoming overweight or obese. Prevalence reaches its peak during the middle-aged years and, once obesity is established, it can be immensely challenging to treat. Few animals start a weight loss program with many of those that doing either failing to reach target weight or rebounding afterwards. As a result, veterinary professionals should focus on prevention of obesity rather than attempting to manage it once it has developed. Veterinary practices should consider establishing a formal program of monitoring body weight and regularly assessing BCS, with strategies tailored to the life stage. As soon as there is evidence of inappropriate weight gain, there should be early intervention with corrective measures. Finally, if an obese animal does successfully lose weight, veterinarians should closely monitor period after weight loss, with regular follow-up weight checks to ensure that bodyweight remains stable. Continuing to feed the therapeutic weight loss diet during the maintenance phase can help to prevent rebound from occurring.

REFERENCES

1. German AJ. The growing problem of obesity in dogs and cats. J Nutr 2006;136: 1940S–6S.
2. Banfield Pet Hospital. State of Pet Health 2012 Report. Available at: www.banfield.com/Banfield/media/PDF/Downloads/soph/Banfield-State-of-Pet-Health-Report_2012.pdf. Accessed January 31, 2016.
3. Mao J, Xia Z, Chen J, et al. Prevalence and risk factors for canine obesity surveyed in veterinary practices in Beijing, China. Prev Vet Med 2012;112: 438–42.
4. Serisier S, Feugier A, Venet C, et al. Faster growth rate in ad libitum-fed cats: a risk factor predicting the likelihood of becoming overweight during adulthood. J Nutr Sci 2013;2:e11.
5. Lund EM, Armstrong PJ, Kirk CA, et al. Prevalence and risk factors for obesity in adult cats from private US veterinary practices. Int J Appl Res Vet Med 2005;3: 88–96.
6. Lund EM, Armstrong PJ, Kirk CA, et al. Prevalence and risk factors for obesity in adult dogs from private US veterinary practices. Int J Appl Res Vet Med 2006;4: 177–86.
7. Reilly JJ, Armstrong J, Dorosty AR, et al. Early life risk factors for obesity in childhood: cohort study. BMJ 2005;330:1357.
8. Haring T, Wichert B, Dolf G, et al. Segregation analysis of overweight body condition in an experimental cat population. J Hered 2011;102(Suppl 1):S28–31.
9. Albuquerque D, Stice E, Rodriguez-Lopez R. Current review of genetics of human obesity: from molecular mechanisms to an evolutionary perspective. Mol Genet Genomics 2015;290:1191–221.
10. Colliard L, Paragon BM, Lemeuet B, et al. Prevalence and risk factors of obesity in an urban population of healthy cats. J Feline Med Surg 2009;11:135–40.
11. Colliard L, Ancel J, Benet JJ, et al. Risk factors for obesity in dogs in France. J Nutr 2006;136:1951S–4S.
12. Flynn MF, Hardie EM, Armstrong PJ. Effect of ovariohysterectomy on maintenance energy requirements in cats. J Am Vet Med Assoc 1996;9:1572–81.

13. Harper EJ, Stack DM, Watson TDG, et al. Effect of feeding regimens on body weight, composition and condition score in cats following ovariohysterectomy. J Small Anim Pract 2001;42:433–8.

14. Heath S. Behaviour problems and welfare. In: Rochlitz I, editor. Feline behavioral medicine. London: Springer; 2005. p. 91–118.

15. Robertson ID. The influence of diet and other factors on owner-perceived obesity in privately owned cats from metropolitan Perth, Western Australia. Prev Vet Med 1999;40:75–93.

16. Allan FJ, Pfeiffer DU, Jones BR, et al. A cross-sectional study of risk factors for obesity in cats in New Zealand. Prev Vet Med 2000;46:183–96.

17. Rowe E, Browne W, Casey R, et al. Risk factors identified for owner-reported feline obesity at around one year of age: dry diet and indoor lifestyle. Prev Vet Med 2015;121:273–81. Available at: http://dx.doi.org/10.1016/j.prevetmed.2015.07.011.

18. Kienzle E, Bergler R, Mandernach A. Comparison of the feeding behavior of the man-animal relationship in owners of normal and obese dogs. J Nutr 1998;128:2779S–82S.

19. Backus RC, Cave NJ, Keisler DH. Gonadectomy and high dietary fat but not high dietary carbohydrate induce gains in body weight and fat of domestic cats. Br J Nutr 2007;98:641–50.

20. Robertson ID. The association of exercise, diet and other factors influence of diet and other factors with owner-perceived obesity in privately owned dogs from metropolitan Perth, Western Australia. Prev Vet Med 1999;58:75–83.

21. Russell K, Sabin R, Holt S, et al. Influence of feeding regimen on body condition in the cat. J Small Anim Pract 2000;41:12–7.

22. Courcier EC, Thompson RM, Mellor DJ. An epidemiological study of environmental factors associated with canine obesity. J Small Anim Pract 2010;51:362–7.

23. Kienzle E, Bergler R. Human-animal relationship of owners of normal and overweight cats. J Nutr 2006;136(Suppl 7):1947S–50S.

24. Weber M, Bissot T, Servet E, et al. A high protein, high fiber diet designed for weight loss improves satiety in dogs. J Vet Intern Med 2007;21:1203–8.

25. Yaissle JE, Holloway C, Buffington CA. Evaluation of owner education as a component of obesity treatment programs for dogs. J Am Vet Med Assoc 2004;224:1932–5.

26. Floerchinger AM, Jackson MI, Jewell DE, et al. Effect of feeding a weight loss food beyond
a caloric restriction period on body composition and resistance to weight gain in dogs. J Am Vet Med Assoc 2015;247:375–84.

27. German AJ, Holden SL, Bissot T, et al. Dietary energy restriction and successful weight loss in obese client-owned dogs. J Vet Intern Med 2007;21:1174–80.

28. German AJ, Holden SL, Bissot T, et al. Changes in body composition during weight loss in obese client-owned cats: Loss of lean tissue mass correlates with overall percentage of weight lost. J Feline Med Surg 2010;10:452–9.

29. German AJ, Titcomb J, Holden SL, et al. Cohort study of the success of controlled weight loss programs for obese dogs. J Vet Intern Med 2015;29:1547–55.

30. Deagle G, Holden SL, Biourge V, et al. The kinetics of weight loss in obese client-owned dogs [abstract]. J Vet Intern Med 2015;29:443–4.

31. Deagle G, Holden SL, Biourge V, et al. The kinetics of weight loss in obese client-owned cats (abstract). Presented at the 58th British Small Animal Veterinary Association Congress. Birmingham, April 8–12, 2015.

32. Mann T, Tomiyama J, Westling E, et al. Medicare's search for effective obesity treatments: diets are not the answer. Am Psychol 2007;62:220–33.

33. German AJ, Holden SL, Morris PJ, et al. Long-term follow-up after weight management in obese dogs: the role of diet in preventing regain. Vet J 2012;192: 65–70.

34. Deagle G, Holden SL, Biourge V, et al. Long-term follow-up after weight management in obese cats. J Nutr Sci 2014;3:e25.

35. Rolph NC, Noble PJM, German AJ. How often do primary care veterinarians record the overweight status of dogs? J Nutr Sci 2014;3:e58.

36. German AJ, Morgan LE. How often do veterinarians assess the bodyweight and body condition of dogs? Vet Rec 2008;163:503–5. Available at: http://veterinaryrecord.bmj.com/content/163/17/503.long.

37. WSAVA Global Nutrition Panel. Nutritional assessment guidelines. Available at: www.wsava.org/sites/default/files/JSAP%20WSAVA%20Global%20Nutritional%20 Assessment%20Guidelines%202011_0.pdf. Accessed January 31, 2016.

38. Witzel AL, Kirk CA, Henry GA, et al. Use of a novel morphometric method and body fat index system for estimation of body composition in overweight and obese dogs. J Am Vet Med Assoc 2014;244:1279–84.

39. Witzel AL, Kirk CA, Henry GA, et al. Use of a morphometric method and body fat index system for estimation of body composition in overweight and obese cats. J Am Vet Med Assoc 2014;244:1285–90.

40. German AJ, Holden SL. Inaccuracy when using tape measures to make zoometric measurements in dogs. J Vet Intern Med 2016;30:418–9.

41. German AJ, Holden SL, Morris PJ, et al. Comparison of a bioimpedance monitor with dual-energy x-ray absorptiometry for noninvasive estimation of percentage body fat in dogs. Am J Vet Res 2010;71:393–8.

42. Raffan E, Holden SL, Cullingham F, et al. Standardized positioning is essential for precise determination of body composition using dual-energy X-ray absorptiometry. J Nutr 2006;136:1976S–8S.

43. Ishioka K, Okumura M, Sagawa M, et al. Computed tomographic assessment of body condition in beagles. Vet Radiol Ultrasound 2005;46:49–53.

44. Bermingham EN, Thomas DG, Morris PJ, et al. Energy requirements of adult cats. Br J Nutr 2010;103:1083–93.

45. Bermingham EN, Thomas DG, Cave NJ, et al. Energy requirements of adult dogs: a meta-analysis. PLoS One 2014;9:e109681.

46. Ballevre O, Anantharaman-Barr G, Gicquello P, et al. Use of the doubly-labeled water method to assess energy expenditure in free living cats and dogs. J Nutr 1994;124:2594S–600S.

47. Scientific Advisory Committee on Nutrition. Reference values for energy. 2011 Available at: www.sacn.gov.uk/reports_position_statements/reports/sacn_ dietary_reference_values_for_energy.html. Accessed January 30, 2014.

48. Walters LM, Ogilvie GK, Salman MD, et al. Repeatability of energy expenditure measurement in clinically normal dogs by use of indirect calorimetry. Am J Vet Res 1993;54:1881–5.

49. German AJ, Holden SL, Mason SL, et al. Imprecision when using measuring cups to weigh out extruded dry kibbled food. J Anim Physiol Anim Nutr 2011;95: 368–73.

50. Wakshlag JJ, Struble AM, Warren BS, et al. Evaluation of dietary energy intake and physical activity in dogs undergoing a controlled weight-loss program. J Am Vet Med Assoc 2012;240:413–9.

51. WHO Multi Centre Reference Study Group. WHO Child Growth Standards based on length/height, weight and age. Acta Paediatr Suppl 2006;450:76–85.

Index

Note: Page numbers of article titles are in **boldface** type.

A

Activity
    as factor in obesity management, 885
Adipokine(s)
    in obesity
        in cats and dogs, 786
        secretion of, 803–804
    in osteoarthritis, 833–834
Adiponectin
    in obesity
        effects of, 820
        secretion of, 803–804
Adipose tissue
    in canine and feline obesity, 786
    normal metabolic function of, 798–799
Adiposity factors
    in maintaining body weight, 775–776
Age
    as factor in obesity, 766
Airway obstruction
    recurrent
        obesity and, 824–826
Asthma
    obesity and, 824

B

Behavior(s)
    as factor in obesity management, 885–892
Biomarker(s)
    weight loss effects on, 820–821
Body weight. *See* Weight
Breed
    as factor in obesity, 764–765

C

Cancer(s)
    obesity and, 846–847
Carbohydrate(s)
    in selecting optimal nutrient profile in weight management in cats
        and dogs, 874

Vet Clin Small Anim 46 (2016) 931–940
http://dx.doi.org/10.1016/S0195-5616(16)30060-2
0195-5616/16/$ – see front matter

Printed and bound by CPI Group (UK) Ltd, Croydon, CR0 4YY

03/10/2024

01040495-0015